CONTENTS
PAGE

THE ALTERNATIVE GREAT GOOD FOOD GUIDE.

When it comes to taking care of our bodies, one of the most important things we can do is to be aware of what we are putting into our bodies. Knowing what's in our food and drinks is essential for maintaining a healthy lifestyle and keeping our bodies functioning properly. In today's world, we have access to a wide variety of food and drinks, many of which contain ingredients that can be harmful to our health. From preservatives and artificial additives to high amounts of sugar and unhealthy fats, it's important to be aware of what's in the products we consume. Knowing which ingredients are beneficial, and which are not, can help us make better choices when it comes to what we put into our bodies. When we're aware of the ingredients in our food and drinks, we can take steps to ensure we're getting the nutrients we need to stay healthy. Eating a balanced diet with a variety of fresh fruits and vegetables, whole grains, lean proteins, and healthy fats is essential for keeping our bodies functioning properly. By knowing what we're consuming, we can make sure we're getting the vitamins and minerals we need to stay healthy. Knowing what we put into our bodies can also help us avoid the negative side effects of certain foods and drinks. Eating too much sugar, for example, can lead to weight gain, diabetes, and other health problems. Knowing which foods contain high amounts of sugar can help us avoid these health risks. Similarly, knowing which foods contain trans fats or other unhealthy ingredients can help us make smarter choices when it comes to our diet. Finally, being aware of what's in our food and drinks can help us make more informed choices about the products we buy. Knowing which items contain healthy ingredients, such as whole grains or fresh vegetables, can help us make better decisions when we're shopping for groceries. And by understanding the labels on products, we can avoid buying items that contain unhealthy ingredients or high amounts of sugar and fat. Overall, it's important to be aware of what we put into our bodies. Knowing which ingredients are beneficial, and which are not, can help us make smarter choices when it comes to our diet. Being aware of the nutrients we consume can help us stay healthy and avoid potential health risks. And understanding what's in the products we buy can help us make more informed decisions when it comes to what we consume.

WHY WE NEED GOOD FOOD

Good food is important for a number of reasons. It is essential for maintaining good health, providing energy, and keeping our bodies nourished. Eating a healthy diet can help to reduce the risk of developing serious health conditions such as obesity, heart disease, and diabetes. Good food can also improve mental health and wellbeing, as it helps to regulate our moods and emotions. Eating a variety of foods can provide us with the essential vitamins, minerals, and other nutrients that our bodies need to function properly. Eating a balanced diet can also help us to maintain a healthy weight. Good food is essential for our overall physical and mental wellbeing

The changes in good diet

Our idea of a good diet changes over time due to a variety of factors, including changes in nutritional science, societal norms, and the emergence of new dietary trends. As nutritional science advances, our understanding of what constitutes a healthy diet evolves, and dietary advice changes in response to new discoveries. For example, the 2015-2020 Dietary Guidelines for Americans recommend a diet that is lower in saturated fat and higher in unsaturated fats, fruits, vegetables, and whole grains than the previous edition of the guidelines. Societal norms also influence our idea of a good diet by influencing what types of foods are perceived as healthy or unhealthy. In the past, certain foods were thought to be unhealthy due to their association with certain cultures or lifestyles; however, today, many of these foods have become more accepted as part of a balanced diet. For example, eggs and avocados are now seen as a nutritious and healthy meal option. The emergence of new dietary trends also affects our idea of a good diet. For example, the popularity of veganism, vegetarianism, and the ketogenic diet has changed the way many people view food. Additionally, the rise of 'clean eating' has led to an emphasis on whole, unprocessed foods as part of a healthy diet. Overall, our idea of a good diet changes over time due to advances in nutritional science, societal norms, and the emergence of new dietary trends. It is important to keep up with the latest dietary advice and to be mindful of the changing perceptions of what constitutes a healthy diet.

Gut Health

Gut health is also another aspect for overall physical and mental wellbeing. The gut is home to trillions of bacteria, viruses and other microorganisms, collectively referred to as the gut microbiota. This microbiota plays a vital role in regulating digestion, immunity, metabolism, and even mental health. The gut microbiome is essential for proper digestion and absorption of nutrients, as well as supporting a healthy digestive system. An unhealthy gut microbiome can lead to digestive disorders such as irritable bowel syndrome, as well as contributing to inflammation and other chronic diseases. The gut microbiome also plays a key role in immunity. The bacteria in the gut can help to strengthen the immune system, as well as helping to protect against infection. An imbalance of gut bacteria can lead to an increased risk of infections and can even affect the body's response to vaccines. The gut microbiome has also been linked to mental health. Research has shown that a healthy gut microbiome can reduce levels of stress, anxiety and depression. An unhealthy gut microbiome can lead to an increase in these mental health issues. Finally, the gut microbiome can affect metabolism. An unhealthy gut microbiome can lead to an increase in fat storage, as well as an increased risk of diabetes and other metabolic disorders. Overall, gut health is incredibly important for physical and mental wellbeing. A healthy gut microbiome is essential for proper digestion and absorption of nutrients, immunity, metabolism, and mental health. Taking steps to maintain a healthy gut microbiome, such as eating a balanced diet, exercising regularly and avoiding processed foods, can help to ensure overall health and wellbeing.

Why has fasting become popular ?

Fasting has become increasingly popular in recent years, with more and more people turning to it to improve their health and wellness. Fasting is the practice of voluntarily abstaining from eating and drinking for a period of time. It is an ancient practice and has been used for centuries for spiritual and religious purposes. The popularity of fasting has grown in recent years as people become aware of its potential health benefits. Research has shown that it can help with weight loss and improve metabolic health. Fasting can also boost energy levels, reduce inflammation, and even help improve mental clarity and focus. Fasting has become popular due to its simplicity and convenience. It eliminates the need to count calories or restrict certain foods. Instead, you simply don't eat or drink anything for a set period of time. This allows people to easily fit fasting into their lifestyle, without needing to make major changes. However it is important that when fasting you still adhere to a good balanced diet. Intermittent fasting is the most popular type of fasting. This involves alternating between periods of eating and fasting, usually in an 8-hour eating window and a 16-hour fasting window. This type of fasting is gaining traction due to its ease of use and effectiveness. Studies have found that it can help with weight loss and reduce the risk of chronic disease. Intermittent fasting is often combined with other health and wellness practices, such as exercise and mindful eating. This helps people to develop healthier habits and create an overall healthier lifestyle. Overall, fasting has become increasingly popular in recent years due to its simplicity and potential health benefits. It is a great way to jumpstart your health journey and make lasting changes. If you are considering trying fasting, it is important to consult a medical professional first to ensure it is safe for you.

Why fasting is so good for you ?

Fasting is a dietary practice that has been used for centuries by many cultures to promote physical, mental, and spiritual health. It is a period of abstaining from all food and beverages, except water. Fasting can have numerous health benefits, including weight loss, improved digestion, increased energy levels, and improved mental clarity. One of the major benefits of fasting is autophagy. Autophagy is a process that happens in our bodies when we fast. It is the natural process of the body breaking down and eliminating damaged cells, proteins, and other waste products. This process is beneficial because it helps prevent the accumulation of damaged cells in the body and reduces the risk of disease. Autophagy also helps to clear out old, damaged proteins and organelles, which can improve cell health. Additionally, fasting can help to improve digestion. When we fast, the body is able to rest from the constant cycle of digestion, allowing the digestive system to heal and repair itself. This helps to improve the efficiency of digestion, leading to better absorption of nutrients from food.

Fasting can also help to regulate hormones.

Fasting can help to balance insulin levels, which can help to reduce cravings, and reduce the risk of diabetes.

In addition, fasting can help to boost the production of growth hormone, which is important for muscle growth and repair.

Fasting can also help to reduce inflammation in the body. Inflammation is a natural process that occurs in response to injury or infection, but too much inflammation can lead to chronic health problems.

It can help to improve mental clarity and focus. Fasting can help to reduce stress levels, which can improve focus and clarity. Overall, fasting is a safe and effective way to improve overall health.

Why Unsaturated fats are now good for the body ?

In recent years, unsaturated fats have been gaining increased attention for their potential health benefits. Unsaturated fats, which include monounsaturated and polyunsaturated fats, are essential dietary fats that are found in a variety of foods such as nuts, seeds, avocados, and some vegetable oils. Unsaturated fats are considered to be "good" fats because they can help to reduce the risk of heart disease and stroke, as well as other health conditions. Monounsaturated fats, also known as "healthy" fats, are found in olive oil, canola oil, and other plant-based oils. They are believed to help reduce cholesterol levels, reduce inflammation, and may even help to protect against certain types of cancer. Polyunsaturated fats, which include omega-3 fatty acids, are found mainly in fatty fish and certain plant-based oils like flaxseed and canola oil. They are known to help reduce the risk of heart disease, stroke, and other cardiovascular diseases. Unsaturated fats are now considered to be beneficial for our overall health because they provide essential fatty acids that our bodies cannot produce on their own. These fatty acids are important for the proper functioning of our cells, organs, and tissues. They also help to reduce inflammation, support healthy blood sugar levels, and promote healthy cholesterol levels. In addition to providing essential fatty acids, unsaturated fats can also help to boost our overall health by providing antioxidants and other beneficial compounds. These compounds are thought to help reduce the risk of certain diseases and protect our cells from damage. Furthermore, unsaturated fats are thought to be beneficial for our mental health, as they are believed to help reduce stress and improve our mood. Overall, unsaturated fats are essential for a healthy diet, and can provide numerous health benefits when consumed in moderation. They are now considered to be "good" fats and are recommended as part of a balanced diet.

The difference between Omega 3 and Omega 6

Omega 3 and omega 6 fatty acids are both essential fatty acids, meaning they are required in the human diet as our bodies cannot produce them. They are both polyunsaturated fats, meaning they have multiple double bonds in the fatty acid chain and are liquid at room temperature. Omega 3 and omega 6 fatty acids have different structures and therefore have different functions. Omega 3 fatty acids are typically found in fish, certain nuts and seeds, and some plants. They are essential for the formation of cell membranes, helping to regulate inflammation in the body and play a role in brain health and development. Omega 6 fatty acids are found in foods like poultry, eggs, and certain vegetable oils. They are important for the formation of prostaglandins, hormone-like molecules that help regulate inflammation and blood clotting. The difference between omega 3 and omega 6 fatty acids is that omega 3 fatty acids are anti-inflammatory, while omega 6 fatty acids are pro-inflammatory. This means that an imbalance between the two can lead to higher levels of inflammation in the body. In general, the ratio of omega 3 to omega 6 fatty acids should be 1:4, with 1 part omega 3 and 4 parts omega 6. Additionally, omega 3 fatty acids are metabolized differently than omega 6 fatty acids, meaning they are less likely to be stored as body fat. This makes them a better option for those looking to lose weight or maintain a healthy weight. Overall, omega 3 and omega 6 fatty acids are both essential for health and should be included in the diet. However, it is important to ensure that the ratio of omega 3 to omega 6 fatty acids is balanced, as an imbalance can lead to higher levels of inflammation in the body.

Why refined sugars are not good ?

Refined sugars, or added sugars, are found in many processed foods and drinks. These sugars, also known as "empty" or "nutrient-poor" calories because they offer no nutritional value, are extremely detrimental to your health. Eating too much of these empty calories can lead to a variety of health issues, such as obesity, diabetes, heart disease, and more. One of the biggest problems with refined sugars is that they are easily and quickly absorbed by the body. This means that, when you consume them, they enter your blood stream rapidly, causing a surge in your blood sugar levels. This can lead to a number of health issues, such as headaches and fatigue, as well as an increased risk of developing diabetes. In addition, refined sugars are addictive. The more you eat, the more you crave them. This can lead to overindulgence and weight gain, as well as an unhealthy reliance on these foods. Refined sugars are also high in calories and low in essential vitamins and minerals. This means that, while they can provide a quick boost of energy, they do not provide any long-term health benefits. In fact, consuming too many refined sugars can actually lead to nutrient deficiencies, which can weaken your immune system and put you at risk for a variety of diseases. Finally, refined sugars can contribute to tooth decay and other dental problems. The bacteria in your mouth break down these sugars, which can lead to plaque build-up and cavities. All in all, refined sugars should be avoided as much as possible. They offer no health benefits and can actually be extremely detrimental to your long-term health. Stick to natural sources of sugar, such as fruits and honey, to ensure that you are getting the vitamins and minerals your body needs.

Good Alternative diets around the world

The Japanese diet is considered one of the healthiest in the world. It is based on a traditional diet that has been around for centuries and consists of foods such as rice, fish, vegetables, seaweed, and soy products. These foods are low in saturated fat and high in healthy proteins, vitamins, and minerals. The Japanese also consume a lot of green tea, which is rich in antioxidants and other beneficial compounds. The Mediterranean diet is another diet that is considered healthy. It is based on the traditional diets of the countries surrounding the Mediterranean Sea and consists of foods such as fresh fruits and vegetables, whole grains, legumes, fish, and healthy fats such as olive oil. This diet is also low in saturated fat and high in beneficial nutrients such as fibre, vitamins, and minerals. The flexitarian diet is a diet that focuses on eating mostly plant-based foods with some animal products added in. This diet is low in saturated fat and high in beneficial nutrients such as fibre, vitamins, and minerals. It is also low in cholesterol and rich in antioxidants.

Alternative diets are becoming increasingly popular around the world. Many people are choosing to omit certain foods from their diets, or completely switch to a different type of diet altogether.

Veganism is a lifestyle that abstains from the use of all animal products and by-products. People who adopt a vegan diet do not consume any animal-based foods, such as eggs, dairy, or honey, and all animal-derived ingredients, such as gelatine, lard, and whey. Instead, vegans get their protein and other nutrients from plant-based sources, including beans, nuts, seeds, fruits, vegetables, and grains. The benefits of a vegan diet are numerous. People who follow a vegan diet tend to have lower body mass index and lower cholesterol levels than those who eat animal products. Vegans also tend to have higher intakes of fibre, magnesium, folate, vitamins C and E, iron, and phytochemicals. Studies have also linked vegan diets with a decreased risk of developing certain cancers, heart disease, diabetes, and obesity. Aside from the health benefits, a vegan diet is also better for the environment. Animal agriculture is a leading contributor to climate change, and the production of animal-based foods requires significantly more resources, such as water and land, than plants. Additionally, it is estimated that a vegan diet can save approximately 1,100 gallons of water per day and reduce greenhouse gas emissions by up to 50%. Adopting a vegan diet can be challenging at first, but there is a wide array of vegan options now available in stores and restaurants. Learning to read labels and becoming familiar with vegan foods and recipes can help to make the transition easier. For those who are just starting out, focusing on eating a variety of fruits, vegetables, whole grains, legumes, nuts, and seeds is a great way to get the nutrients needed for a healthy diet.

The raw food diet is a dietary approach that is based on the consumption of uncooked and unprocessed plant-based foods. This diet is becoming increasingly popular as more people are becoming aware of the nutritional and health benefits of eating raw foods. The idea behind the raw food diet is to maximize the natural nutrients and enzymes found in plant-based foods. By consuming these foods in their natural, unprocessed state, the body is able to absorb and utilize the nutrients more effectively. This helps to promote overall health, leading to increased energy, improved digestion, and a stronger immune system. In addition to providing essential nutrients, raw food diets can also provide a number of other benefits. Studies have shown that consuming raw foods can help to reduce cholesterol levels, improve cardiovascular health, and even lower the risk of certain types of cancer. Additionally, raw foods are typically high in fibre, which can help to keep the digestive system functioning optimally. The raw food diet typically excludes any food that has been cooked or heated above 116°F. This means that all grains, legumes, and most dairy products are off-limits. Additionally, processed foods, refined sugars, and artificial additives should be avoided. Instead, the raw food diet focuses on fresh fruits and vegetables, nuts, seeds, and sprouted grains. These foods are usually consumed either raw or lightly steamed and can be eaten in their whole form or blended into smoothies or juices. Although the raw food diet may have health benefits, there are also some potential drawbacks. For instance, some raw food diets are low in protein, and may not provide enough of this essential nutrient for some individuals. Additionally, consuming raw foods can also increase the risk of food-borne illness, so it's important to be mindful of food safety practices when preparing raw foods. Overall, the raw food diet is a healthy and nutritious way to eat. If you're considering making the switch to a raw food diet, it's important to speak with your doctor or a nutritionist to ensure that you're getting all the essential nutrients your body needs.

The Paleo diet is a nutrition plan that advocates eating the same foods that were consumed by our early ancestors during the Palaeolithic era. This diet focuses on nutrient-dense, unprocessed, whole foods such as fresh fruits, vegetables, eggs, nuts, seeds, and lean animal proteins. The Paleo diet eliminates dairy, grains, legumes, refined sugars, processed foods, and trans fats, as these foods were not available during the Palaeolithic era. Proponents of the Paleo diet claim that it can reduce inflammation, improve digestion, and promote weight loss. The diet is also thought to reduce the risk of chronic diseases such as heart disease, diabetes, and cancer by eliminating processed foods from the diet. Additionally, the diet emphasizes eating nutrient-dense foods that are high in vitamins, minerals, and antioxidants. The Paleo diet is a great way to reduce your calorie intake and improve overall health. It is important to note that the Paleo diet is not a weight-loss diet and should not be used as a replacement for a balanced, nutrient-rich diet. Instead, the Paleo diet should be used as a supplement to an already healthy diet. In addition to eating a nutrient-dense diet, it is important to get regular physical activity. Exercise can help improve your mood, reduce stress, and enhance your overall health. If you are considering trying the Paleo diet, it is important to consult with your healthcare provider before beginning to ensure that it is the right choice for you.

Gluten free diets are becoming increasingly popular among individuals looking to improve their health. Gluten-free foods are free of the protein gluten, which is found in wheat, barley, and rye. Individuals who have an intolerance to gluten, or those diagnosed with celiac disease, must follow a strict gluten-free diet. A gluten-free diet is beneficial for those with gluten intolerance, as it eliminates the symptoms caused by consuming gluten. Symptoms of gluten intolerance can range from mild discomfort to severe reactions, and can include bloating, diarrhoea, nausea, and fatigue. Following a gluten-free diet can help to reduce or even eliminate these symptoms. When following a gluten-free diet, individuals should focus on eating nutrient-dense foods such as fresh fruits and vegetables, lean meats, fish, nuts and seeds, and gluten-free grains such as quinoa, amaranth, and buckwheat. Eating a variety of foods will help to ensure that individuals get the vitamins, minerals, and other nutrients they need for optimal health. Eating gluten-free can also be an enjoyable experience. There is a wide selection of gluten-free products available at most grocery stores, and many restaurants now offer gluten-free options. Additionally, there are many delicious recipes available online. With a bit of planning and experimentation, individuals can still enjoy a wide variety of delicious meals while following a gluten-free diet.

Overall, following a gluten-free diet can be an effective way to improve health and reduce symptoms of gluten intolerance. By making sure to eat a wide variety of nutrient-dense foods and experimenting with recipes, individuals can make following a gluten-free diet a positive and enjoyable experience.

The ketogenic diet is a high-fat, low-carbohydrate diet that has become increasingly popular in recent years. It has been used to treat a variety of health conditions, including epilepsy, diabetes, and obesity. The diet works by drastically reducing the number of carbohydrates consumed and replacing them with high amounts of healthy fats. The goal of the diet is to put the body into a state of ketosis, which is a natural metabolic state where the body burns fat instead of carbohydrates for energy. The ketogenic diet consists of eating mostly healthy fats, moderate amounts of protein, and very few carbohydrates. The amount of carbohydrates consumed should be kept to a minimum, usually about 5-10% of total daily calories. It's important to note that the body needs some carbohydrates to function properly, so even on a ketogenic diet, it's important to consume some complex carbohydrates, such as vegetables and fruits. In general, the ketogenic diet has been found to be beneficial for a variety of health conditions, including diabetes, obesity, and epilepsy. It has also been found to help reduce inflammation, improve cholesterol levels, and even help with weight loss. When beginning a ketogenic diet, it's important to begin slowly and gradually increase the amount of healthy fats consumed. It's also important to make sure to get enough electrolytes, such as potassium, magnesium, and sodium, which can become depleted on the diet. Additionally, it's important to get adequate amounts of vitamins, minerals, and other nutrients through foods. Overall, the ketogenic diet is a healthy alternative to traditional diets that can have beneficial effects on a variety of health conditions. It's important to be mindful of the foods consumed and to make sure to get enough electrolytes, vitamins, and minerals. It's also important to consult a doctor before beginning any new diet.

These are just a few of the alternative diets that people are choosing around the world. Each one has its own unique benefits and may work better for some people than others. Each diet has its own set of benefits and drawbacks, so it is important to do your research and discuss it with your doctor before making any drastic changes. It is important to find a diet that works for you and your lifestyle, and to make sure you are getting all the nutrients you need.

THE "BIG 3" MACRONUTRIENTS (MACROS)

Proteins

Proteins are essential macromolecules that make up the building blocks of all living things. They are organic molecules that contain carbon, hydrogen, oxygen, and nitrogen and are made up of amino acids. Proteins are essential for the structure, function, and regulation of the body's tissues and organs. Proteins are responsible for countless tasks throughout the body. They are involved in the structure of cells, muscles, and organs, as well as in enzymatic reactions, hormone production, and transportation of molecules across cell membranes. Proteins can also be used as a fuel source, providing energy in the form of calories. The body needs protein to repair tissues, create hormones, and make enzymes and other chemicals. Protein is also necessary for growth and development, as well as for the maintenance of bones, muscles, skin, and other tissues. Protein can be found in a variety of foods, including meat, fish, eggs, dairy products, legumes, nuts, and seeds. The recommended daily intake of protein for an adult is 0.8 grams of protein for every kilogram of body weight. A diet that includes a variety of protein-rich foods can help ensure adequate protein intake. In addition to dietary sources, protein supplements can be used to increase protein intake. Protein supplements come in many forms, including powders, shakes, and bars. The type of protein supplement chosen should depend on individual needs and goals. Proteins are essential macromolecules that make up the building blocks of all living things. They are involved in the structure, function, and regulation of the body's tissues and organs, and they provide energy in the form of calories. Protein can be found in a variety of foods, as well as in protein supplements. Adequate protein intake is essential for growth and development, as well as for the maintenance of bones, muscles, skin, and other tissues.

Proteins are essential nutrients for the human body. They are the building blocks of life. Proteins are made up of amino acids, which are the building blocks of proteins. Protein helps to build and repair muscles, bones, skin, and other body tissues. It also helps to make hormones and enzymes. Proteins play a key role in many bodily processes, including cell growth and repair, hormone production, energy production, and metabolism. They also help to keep the immune system functioning properly. In addition, proteins can help to reduce hunger and provide energy for physical activity. Proteins are essential for muscle growth and development. When you exercise, your muscles break down and rebuild themselves. Protein helps to rebuild the muscle tissue and make it stronger. Eating a diet that is high in protein can help to build and maintain muscle mass. Proteins are also important for healthy bones. When calcium and phosphorus combine with protein, they create a substance called hydroxyapatite, which helps to form the framework for bones. Without enough protein in the diet, bones become weak and prone to fractures. Proteins are also important for healthy skin. When skin cells break down, proteins help to rebuild them. Proteins also help to create collagen and elastin, which are essential components of healthy skin. Proteins are important for a healthy immune system. Proteins can help the body fight off infection by producing antibodies that help to identify and destroy harmful bacteria and viruses. Finally, proteins are important for healthy brain function. Proteins can help to produce neurotransmitters, which are chemicals responsible for communication between brain cells. This helps to keep the brain functioning properly. In conclusion, proteins are essential nutrients that are important for many bodily processes. They help to build and repair muscle, bones, skin, and other body tissues. They also help to regulate hormones and enzymes, reduce hunger, and provide energy for physical activity. Eating a diet that is high in protein can help to keep the body healthy and functioning properly.

The best food sources for protein

Protein is one of the most important macronutrients for a person's health. It helps build and repair muscle, aids in digestion, and provides energy. But with so many different protein sources available, it can be difficult to know which one is best for you. Here are some of the best food sources for protein:

Lean Meats: Lean meats are one of the most popular sources of protein, especially for those following a low-fat diet. Lean meats are an excellent source of essential amino acids, the building blocks of all proteins. Lean meats are also low in fat and calories and can help to reduce your risk of obesity, heart disease, and diabetes. Lean meats are a great source of complete proteins, meaning they contain all the essential amino acids your body needs. These proteins are easily digested and broken down, allowing your body to absorb the nutrients quickly and easily. Lean meats are also high in B vitamins, which are essential for your body to use energy and process nutrients. Lean meats are also very low in fat and calories, making them a great choice for those looking to lose weight. They are also low in cholesterol, which can help to lower your risk of heart disease, stroke, and other cardiovascular diseases. Additionally, lean meats are low in saturated fat, which can help reduce your risk of type 2 diabetes. Overall, lean meats are an excellent source of protein and can help you meet your daily protein requirements. They are low in fat, calories, and cholesterol, making them a great choice for those looking to improve their health and reduce their risk of obesity, heart disease, and diabetes. Lean meats are also an excellent source of essential amino acids, B vitamins, and other essential nutrients, making them an ideal choice for those looking to get the most out of their diet.

Eggs: Eggs are a powerhouse of nutrition, and they are one of the best sources of protein available. Studies have shown that eating eggs can help with weight loss, muscle building, and a healthier overall diet. Protein is essential for our bodies to function, and eggs can be a great source of it. Eggs are made up of about 10-13% protein, and all the essential amino acids our body needs. The egg white contains the majority of the protein, and the yolk contains the cholesterol and fat. Eggs are also an excellent source of many other important vitamins and minerals. They contain vitamins A, D, E, and K, as well as folate, iron, calcium, phosphorus, and potassium. They are also full of antioxidants, which help protect against damage from free radicals. Eggs are also relatively low in calories, with only about 80 calories per whole egg. This makes them an ideal option for people who are trying to lose weight or maintain their weight. Eating eggs can also help with muscle building. Eggs are a complete source of protein, meaning they contain all the essential amino acids that your body needs to build and repair muscle. Eating eggs can also help you feel full and satisfied for longer, which can help with weight loss. Finally, eggs are a great source of healthy fats. The yolk is full of healthy fatty acids, such as omega-3 fatty acids, which can help reduce inflammation and cholesterol levels. In conclusion, eggs are an excellent source of protein, vitamins, minerals, and healthy fats. They are low in calories, and can help with weight loss, muscle building, and overall health. For these reasons, eggs are a great addition to any healthy diet.

Fish: Fish are an excellent source of protein and other essential nutrients. They are a low-fat source of protein and contain high amounts of omega-3 fatty acids, which are beneficial for health. Fish are also a great source of vitamins and minerals, including vitamin D, vitamin A, selenium, and iodine, as well as zinc, iron, and magnesium. Fish are also a great source of healthy fats and essential amino acids, which are the building blocks for protein. Fish are a good source of essential fatty acids, such as EPA and DHA, which are beneficial for heart health. Fish are also an excellent source of B vitamins, including vitamin B12, which is important for energy and healthy brain function. In addition to being a great source of protein, fish are also high in other beneficial nutrients. They are a great source of calcium, phosphorus, and potassium, which are essential for bone and muscle health. They are also high in selenium, an important antioxidant, and zinc, which is important for a healthy immune system. Fish are also a great source of omega-3 fatty acids, which are beneficial for reducing inflammation and reducing the risk of heart disease and stroke. Omega-3 fatty acids are also important for brain health and cognitive function. Overall, fish are an excellent source of protein and essential nutrients. They are a low-fat source of protein and contain high amounts of omega-3 fatty acids, which are beneficial for health. Fish are also a great source of vitamins and minerals, including vitamin D, vitamin A, selenium, and iodine, as well as zinc, iron, and magnesium. They are also a great source of essential fatty acids, such as EPA and DHA, which are beneficial for heart health. Thus, fish are a great source of protein and other essential nutrients, making them an important part of a healthy diet.

Nuts and Seeds: Nuts and seeds are a great source of protein and other nutrients. They are packed full of healthy fats, vitamins, minerals, and amino acids, making them an excellent choice for those looking to get more protein in their diet. Nuts and seeds are a great source of plant-based protein. They are particularly high in protein compared to other plant-based foods, with some varieties providing up to 7g of protein per 30g serving. They also provide essential fatty acids, minerals, and vitamins that are essential for good health. For example, almonds are a good source of dietary fibre, vitamin E, magnesium, phosphorus, and manganese. Nuts and seeds are easy to incorporate into your diet, making them a convenient and versatile source of protein. They can be eaten as a snack, added to salads, and used as a topping on yogurt or oatmeal. They can also be ground up into nut butter or blended into smoothies. The health benefits of nuts and seeds extend beyond just the protein content. They are also a good source of healthy fats, antioxidants, and fibre. Nuts and seeds are low in calories and fat and can help you to feel fuller for longer, which can help to reduce cravings and overeating. Nuts and seeds are a great source of protein and other essential nutrients. They are easy to incorporate into your diet and provide a range of health benefits. If you're looking to increase your protein intake, nuts and seeds are an excellent choice.

Dairy: Dairy is an incredibly nutrient-dense food source, providing a variety of essential vitamins and minerals, as well as being a great source of protein. Dairy products are a great way to get your daily protein requirements, and they can be included in a variety of meals and snacks. Protein is an essential nutrient that helps build and repair muscle, skin, and bones. It also helps maintain healthy blood sugar levels and is important for hormone production. Protein found in dairy is considered a complete protein source because it contains all nine essential amino acids. This means it can be easily and quickly used by the body. In addition to protein, dairy contains a variety of other essential nutrients. Dairy is a good source of calcium, which is important for strong bones and teeth. It also contains phosphorus, vitamin A, and vitamin D, which are all important for overall health. Dairy also contains beneficial fatty acids and is a good source of B vitamins. Furthermore, dairy is an easy and convenient way to get your daily dose of protein. It can be enjoyed in a variety of ways, from adding it to a smoothie or yogurt parfait to having a glass of milk with a meal. Dairy products can also be used as a substitute for meat in many recipes, making it a great option for those looking to reduce their meat intake. In conclusion, dairy is an excellent source of protein and other essential nutrients. It is an easy and convenient way to get your daily dose of protein, and it can be incorporated into a variety of meals and snacks. Dairy can also be used as a substitute for meat in many recipes, making it a great choice for those looking to reduce their meat intake.

Beans and Legumes: Beans and Legumes are an excellent source of protein, particularly for those who don't eat animal products. They are an essential part of any healthy diet, providing essential amino acids, minerals, and vitamins. Protein is essential for the growth and maintenance of our bodies. It plays a role in building and repairing muscle and tissue, producing enzymes and hormones, and facilitating the transport of nutrients. Beans and legumes are a great source of protein, containing between 7 and 25 grams of protein per cup. They are also a good source of fibre, providing between 5 and 10 grams of fibre per cup. This makes them a great addition to any diet as they can help to reduce cholesterol and improve digestive health. Additionally, they are low in fat and provide essential vitamins and minerals such as iron, magnesium, and zinc. For those on a plant-based diet, beans and legumes are an excellent source of protein. They are also a great source of plant-based iron, which is essential for the production of haemoglobin, the molecule responsible for transporting oxygen in the blood. For vegetarians, legumes are a great source of vitamin B12, which is essential for cell metabolism. Beans and legumes are also a great source of complex carbohydrates, which provide energy and help to regulate blood sugar levels. Additionally, they are a great source of antioxidants, which can help to protect against free radical damage and reduce inflammation. Overall, beans and legumes are a great source of protein, fibre, vitamins, minerals, and antioxidants. They are an essential part of any healthy diet and are incredibly versatile, making them a great addition to any meal. Whether you're vegetarian, vegan, or just trying to eat healthier, beans and legumes are a great way to get the protein and nutrients you need.

Quinoa:

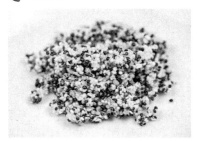

Write a detailed piece on why quinoa is a good source for protein Quinoa is an ancient grain that has become increasingly popular in recent years due to its versatility, nutritional value and health benefits. It is a complete source of protein, meaning that it contains all nine essential amino acids. Quinoa is also high in fibre, which can help to regulate blood sugar levels and can aid in digestion. Additionally, quinoa contains vitamins and minerals such as iron, magnesium, phosphorus and zinc as well as antioxidants. Quinoa is relatively easy to prepare and can be eaten as a side dish, added to salads or made into a porridge. It is also gluten-free, making it a great alternative for those with gluten sensitivities. Quinoa is a good source of plant-based protein and can help to meet the daily protein requirements for vegetarians and vegans. It is also a great source of energy, providing a slow release of carbohydrates that can help to sustain energy levels throughout the day. Due to its high protein content, quinoa can help to promote muscle growth and repair. It can also help to support a healthy immune system and can promote healthy skin, hair and nails due to its high levels of essential amino acids and minerals. Additionally, quinoa can help to reduce cholesterol levels and can aid in weight loss due to its low-calorie and high-fibre content. Overall, quinoa is an excellent source of plant-based protein and is packed with essential vitamins and minerals. The wide range of health benefits it provides makes it an excellent choice for those looking to increase their intake of plant-based proteins.

Soy: Soy is an excellent source of protein, and it's quickly becoming a popular choice for those looking to increase their protein intake. Soy is a plant-based protein, which makes it a great alternative to animal proteins like beef, chicken, and fish. Soy is also a complete protein, meaning it contains all of the essential amino acids our bodies need. One of the reasons soy is a great source of protein is that it contains essential fatty acids. These fatty acids help regulate our hormones, protect our cells from damage, and even improve our moods. Soy also contains both soluble and insoluble fibre, which helps keep our digestion regular and our cholesterol levels healthy. Soy is low in saturated fat, so it's a great choice for those who are trying to watch their calorie intake. One cup of cooked soybeans contains approximately 28 grams of protein, so you're getting a solid amount of protein with just one serving. Soy is also low in calories and high in essential vitamins and minerals, so it's a good choice for those looking to maintain a healthy weight. Soy is also a great source of antioxidants, which help protect our bodies from oxidative stress and damage. Antioxidants can help reduce inflammation and protect our cells from damage caused by free radicals. Soy is also a good source of phytochemicals, which can help reduce the risk of certain cancers and other diseases. Overall, soy is an excellent source of protein. Not only is it a complete protein, but it's also low in saturated fat, high in fibre, and loaded with essential vitamins and minerals. Soy is also a great source of antioxidants and phytochemicals, which can help protect our bodies from oxidative stress and reduce the risk of certain diseases. If you're looking for a plant-based source of protein, soy is definitely worth considering.

By including a variety of these foods in your diet, you can ensure that you are getting all the protein you need to stay healthy. Eating a balanced diet that includes protein-rich foods is the key to good health.

Why having too much is not good

Eating too much protein can be detrimental to your health. Excessive protein intake can cause dehydration, weight gain, kidney problems, and even cancer. The human body needs protein to repair and build cells, and to make hormones, enzymes, and other body chemicals. Proteins also provide energy and help carry oxygen throughout the body. The daily recommended intake of protein is 0.8 grams of protein per kilogram of body weight. This means that for a person who weighs 70 kilograms, the recommended daily intake would be 56 grams of protein. However, eating too much protein can have a number of adverse effects on the body. Excess protein can lead to dehydration. The body needs water to digest and process proteins, so when too much protein is consumed, it can cause the body to become dehydrated. This can lead to headaches, fatigue, and difficulty concentrating. Eating too much protein can also cause weight gain. This is because proteins are calorie-dense, meaning they contain a lot of calories in a small amount of food. When eaten in excess, these calories can lead to weight gain. Additionally, the body stores excess protein as fat, which can increase your risk of obesity and other health problems. Excessive protein intake can also cause kidney problems. The kidneys are responsible for filtering waste products from the body, and when too much protein is consumed, it can put a strain on the kidneys, leading to kidney stones, kidney failure, and other kidney-related problems. Finally, excessive protein intake has been linked to an increased risk of some types of cancer. Studies have found that eating too much protein can cause an increase in the production of certain hormones, which can increase the risk of developing certain types of cancer, such as breast and prostate cancer. Therefore, it is important to consume the recommended daily amount of protein in order to stay healthy. The recommended daily amount of protein is 0.8 grams of protein per kilogram of body weight. Eating too much protein can lead to a number of health problems, so it is important to stick to the recommended daily amount.

Carbohydrates

Carbohydrates, or "carbs" for short, are one of the three main macronutrients, along with proteins and fats. Carbs are the body's main source of energy, and they play an important role in a healthy diet. Carbs are found in a variety of foods, including fruits, vegetables, grains, legumes, dairy products, and sugars. While all of these foods contain some form of carbs, they are not all the same. Some carbs are simple, meaning they are quickly broken down and absorbed by the body, while others are complex and take longer to digest. Simple carbs are found in foods like fruits, vegetables, and dairy products. These carbs are typically made up of one or two sugar molecules, such as glucose and fructose. Simple carbs are quickly broken down and absorbed by the body, providing energy quickly. Complex carbs, on the other hand, are made up of more than two sugar molecules linked together. They are found in foods like grains, legumes, and some vegetables. Complex carbs take longer to digest, and they provide energy over a longer period of time. Carbs are an important part of a healthy diet, as they provide the body with energy. They are also essential for proper brain and muscle function. Carbs should make up 45-65% of a person's daily calories, and it is important to focus on complex carbs, such as whole grains and legumes, rather than simple carbs, such as sugars and processed foods. In conclusion, carbohydrates are one of the three main macronutrients, and they are an important part of a healthy diet. They provide the body with energy, and they are essential for proper brain and muscle function. It is important to focus on complex carbs, such as whole grains and legumes, rather than simple carbs, such as sugars and processed foods.

Carbs are an important and necessary part of a healthy diet. They provide energy, help build strong muscles, and are essential for proper brain function. Carbs are the body's main source of energy. When you eat carbs, your body breaks them down into glucose, which is then used as fuel for your muscles and brain. Without carbs, your body would not be able to perform at its best. Carbs are also essential for building strong muscles. When you exercise, your body breaks down muscle tissue, which is then rebuilt using the glucose from carbs. Without adequate amounts of carbs, your body would not have the energy to rebuild those muscles. Carbs are also necessary for proper brain function. Glucose is the primary fuel for your brain, so without carbs, your brain would be unable to function properly. Finally, carbs are important for maintaining a healthy weight. Eating the right kinds of carbs can help you maintain a healthy weight and prevent obesity. Foods that are high in carbs, such as fruits, vegetables, and whole grains, are low in calories and can help you feel full longer. So, while carbs may have gotten a bad reputation over the years, they are actually an important part of a healthy diet. Eating the right kinds of carbs can help you maintain a healthy weight, build strong muscles, and keep your brain functioning properly.

The best food sources for carbohydrates

Carbohydrates are an essential part of a balanced diet and provide the body with its main source of energy. The best food sources for carbohydrates are those that are high in fibre, contain complex carbohydrates, and are low in added sugars. Whole grains are a great source of complex carbohydrates and fibre. They contain essential vitamins and minerals and are digested more slowly than other carbohydrates.

Beans, peas and lentils: Beans, peas and lentils are a great source of carbohydrates and offer many health benefits. They are a nutrient-dense food, meaning they are low in calories but high in essential vitamins and minerals. They are also high in fibre, which helps to keep us feeling full for longer and helps to regulate blood sugar levels. Beans, peas and lentils are also a great source of complex carbohydrates. Complex carbohydrates are broken down slowly by the body, providing a steady source of energy for hours after eating. This helps to keep us feeling full for longer periods of time, reducing the likelihood of snacking between meals. In addition to the dietary benefits, beans, peas and lentils are also a great source of plant-based proteins. They are an excellent source of protein for vegans and vegetarians, and they provide a healthy alternative to meat-based proteins. They are also low in saturated fats and contain no cholesterol, making them a healthier choice overall. Beans, peas and lentils are also a great source of antioxidants. Antioxidants help to protect the body from damage caused by free radicals, which can lead to chronic disease. Antioxidants can also help to reduce inflammation in the body, which is linked to many chronic diseases. Finally, beans, peas and lentils are very versatile and can be used in a variety of recipes. They can be used to make soups, salads, stews, and casseroles. They can also be used as a side dish or as a main course. In conclusion, beans, peas and lentils are a great source of complex carbohydrates, proteins, and antioxidants. Not only are they nutrient-dense and low in calories, but they are also very versatile and can be used in a variety of recipes. For these reasons, beans, peas and lentils are an excellent choice for a healthy and balanced diet.

Fruits and vegetables: Fruits and vegetables are an excellent source of carbohydrates, as they are packed with essential vitamins, minerals, and dietary fibre. Carbohydrates provide the body with energy and are necessary for a healthy diet. Fruits and vegetables are some of the most nutrient-dense foods available, and they are a great choice for those looking to increase their carbohydrate intake. Fruits and vegetables are rich sources of complex carbohydrates, which are made up of long chains of sugar molecules. These carbohydrates provide the body with slow-burning energy, helping to keep you feeling full for longer and providing a steady supply of fuel throughout the day. Complex carbohydrates are also beneficial for maintaining a healthy gut microbiome, as they are a great source of dietary fibre. Fibre helps to promote healthy digestion and can also help reduce the risk of certain diseases, including type 2 diabetes and heart disease. Fruits and vegetables also contain simple carbohydrates, which are made up of shorter chains of sugar molecules. These types of carbohydrates provide the body with quick bursts of energy, making them ideal for fuelling physical activity. Simple carbohydrates are also a great source of essential vitamins and minerals, including potassium, magnesium, and iron. In addition to providing energy, fruits and vegetables are also an important source of antioxidants. Antioxidants help to protect the body from free radical damage, which can lead to chronic diseases such as cancer, heart disease, and Alzheimer's. They also help to reduce inflammation, which can help to improve overall health and wellness. Overall, fruits and vegetables are an excellent source of carbohydrates and should be a staple of any healthy diet. They are packed with essential vitamins, minerals, and dietary fibre, and provide the body with slow-burning energy and quick bursts of fuel. They are also a great source of antioxidants, which can help protect the body from free radical damage and reduce inflammation. Fruits and vegetables are a great choice for those looking to increase their carbohydrate intake in a healthy and nutritious way.

Dairy: Diary products are a great source of carbohydrates and provide many essential nutrients in the diet. They are very versatile and can be enjoyed in a variety of ways. Dairy products are an excellent source of carbohydrates, providing energy and essential nutrients. They are a great source of high-quality protein, which helps to build and maintain muscle mass. Dairy products also provide several essential vitamins and minerals, including calcium, phosphorus, magnesium, and zinc. These nutrients are important for bone health, and for proper functioning of the body's organs and systems. Not only are dairy products a great source of carbohydrates, but they are also convenient and easy to incorporate into meals. You can enjoy dairy products in numerous ways, including in smoothies, yogurt, cheese, and milk. Dairy products can also be used to create tasty and nutritious snacks, such as cheese and crackers, or yogurt and fruit. Dairy products can also help to regulate blood sugar, as they contain a combination of simple and complex carbohydrates. This helps to keep your energy levels steady throughout the day and helps to prevent sharp spikes and dips in blood sugar. In addition, dairy products contain beneficial bacteria, known as probiotics, which help to promote digestive health. Studies have also shown that consuming dairy products regularly can help to reduce the risk of developing certain diseases, such as heart disease and type 2 diabetes. Overall, dairy products are a great source of carbohydrates and essential nutrients and can be enjoyed in a variety of ways. They are convenient, easy to incorporate into meals, and can help to regulate blood sugar and promote digestive health.

Nuts and seeds: Nuts and seeds are a great source of carbohydrates and other essential nutrients. They are packed with complex carbohydrates, dietary fibre, vitamins, minerals, and healthy fats. Eating nuts and seeds daily can help to provide your body with the energy it needs to function properly. Complex carbohydrates found in nuts and seeds provide long-lasting energy that can help you stay full for longer. They contain fibre, which helps to slow the digestion process and helps to keep your blood sugar levels steady. Eating nuts and seeds can also help to reduce risk of chronic diseases like heart disease, diabetes, and obesity. Nuts and seeds are also rich in vitamins and minerals. They are an excellent source of vitamin E, which helps to protect the body from oxidative damage and can help to prevent certain types of cancer. They are also a great source of folate, which helps to support a healthy pregnancy and can help to reduce the risk of birth defects. In addition, nuts and seeds are full of healthy fats. Many of the fatty acids found in nuts and seeds are unsaturated, which helps to reduce bad cholesterol levels and can help to reduce the risk of heart disease. Finally, nuts and seeds are a great source of plant-based protein. Eating nuts and seeds can provide your body with all the essential amino acids it needs to build and repair muscle tissue. Overall, nuts and seeds are an excellent source of carbohydrates, dietary fibre, vitamins, minerals, and healthy fats. Eating nuts and seeds daily can provide your body with long-lasting energy and help to reduce the risk of chronic diseases. They are also a great source of plant-based protein and can help to support a healthy pregnancy.

Whole grain breads and pastas: Whole grains are a great source of carbohydrates, and they provide many health benefits. Whole grains are packed with fibre, vitamins, minerals, and essential fatty acids that are important for optimal health. They are also low in calories and fat, and high in protein, making them a great choice for those looking to lose weight. Whole grains are complex carbohydrates, meaning they are slowly digested and absorbed into the bloodstream. This helps to regulate blood sugar levels and provide sustained energy throughout the day. Whole grains are also a great source of B vitamins, which are essential for energy production and metabolism. Eating whole grains can help to reduce the risk of chronic diseases such as heart disease, stroke, and Type 2 diabetes. Whole grains can also help to reduce inflammation in the body, which can lead to many health conditions such as arthritis and autoimmune diseases. Whole grains also provide other important nutrients such as magnesium, zinc, and iron. These nutrients are essential for a healthy immune system and can help to protect against certain types of cancer. Eating whole grains can also help to promote digestive health. The high fibre content helps to keep the digestive system running smoothly and can help to reduce the risk of constipation, bloating, and other digestive issues. Whole grains can also help to reduce cholesterol levels. Whole grains breads and pastas are an excellent source of carbohydrates and provide a variety of health benefits. They are low in calories and fat, high in fibre and protein, and provide essential vitamins, minerals, and fatty acids. Eating whole grains can help to reduce the risk of chronic diseases, reduce inflammation, and promote digestive health. For these reasons, whole grains breads and pastas are an excellent choice for those looking to improve their overall health.

In conclusion, the best food sources of carbohydrates are those that are high in fibre, contain complex carbohydrates, and are low in added sugars. Whole grains, legumes, fruits and vegetables, dairy products, nuts and seeds, and whole grain breads and pastas are all excellent sources of carbohydrates.

Why having too much is not good

Having too many carbs is not good for your health. Eating too many carbs can lead to weight gain, high blood sugar levels, and even diabetes. Carbs are the main source of energy for the body. They provide fuel for physical activity and brain function. However, when you consume too many carbs, your body can't process them all and stores the extra as fat. This can lead to weight gain. High levels of carbs in the blood can also be harmful. Too much glucose in the blood can lead to insulin resistance, which is a precursor to type 2 diabetes. Insulin is a hormone that helps regulate blood sugar levels. If your body becomes resistant to insulin, it won't be able to properly process the carbs in your diet. This can lead to elevated blood sugar levels, which can damage your blood vessels, nerves, and organs. Eating too many carbs can also cause other health issues. They can increase your risk of heart disease and stroke, as well as increase your risk of developing certain types of cancer. Additionally, eating too many carbs can lead to indigestion and other digestive issues. Overall, it is important to limit your intake of carbs as part of a healthy diet. Try to focus on eating complex carbs such as whole grains, fruits, vegetables, and legumes. These types of carbs provide the body with essential vitamins and minerals without the excess calories and fat that come from processed and refined carbs. Eating a balanced diet and limiting your intake of carbs can help you maintain a healthy weight and reduce your risk of chronic diseases.

Fats

Fats are an essential part of a healthy diet and are found in many foods. Fats are made up of triglycerides which are molecules composed of three fatty acids attached to a glycerol backbone. Fats are an important source of energy and provide essential fatty acids which are not made by the body and must be obtained through food. Fats are also important for absorbing certain vitamins and other nutrients, and for protecting organs and maintaining cell membranes. Fats can be divided into two main categories: saturated and unsaturated. Saturated fats are solid at room temperature and are typically found in animal products such as red meat, poultry, and dairy products. Unsaturated fats are liquid at room temperature and are typically found in plant sources such as nuts, seeds, and vegetable oils. Saturated fats are typically solid at room temperature and should be limited in the diet because they can increase the risk of heart disease. Unsaturated fats are typically liquid at room temperature and can be beneficial for heart health when consumed in moderation. Trans fats are a type of unsaturated fat that is created through a process called hydrogenation. Trans fats are typically found in processed foods and should be avoided as they increase the risk of heart disease. When choosing fats, it is important to focus on unsaturated fats, such as those found in nuts, seeds, vegetable oils, and fish. It is also important to limit the intake of saturated fats and trans fats. Eating a diet that is rich in unsaturated fats can help to reduce the risk of heart disease, while also providing essential fatty acids and other nutrients.

Fats provide our bodies with energy, help us absorb certain vitamins and minerals, and are necessary for proper brain and nerve function. Although fats have been demonized in the past, research now shows that the right kinds of fats can actually be beneficial for our health. One of the main benefits of fats is that they provide our bodies with energy. Fats are a concentrated form of energy and provide more than twice the energy per gram than carbohydrates and proteins. This makes them an important source of fuel for our bodies, especially during periods of exertion. In addition to providing us with energy, fats also help our bodies absorb certain vitamins and minerals. Vitamins A, D, E, and K are all fat-soluble vitamins, meaning that they require fat to be absorbed into our bodies. Without enough fat, our bodies cannot properly absorb these important vitamins and minerals. Fats also help us absorb carotenoids, which are important antioxidants that can help protect against disease. Finally, fats are essential for proper brain and nerve function. Our brains are made up of mostly fat, and certain types of fat are important for proper brain development. Fats are also important for the transmission of nerve signals, allowing our brains to communicate with the rest of our bodies. In conclusion, fats are an essential part of a healthy diet and are important for providing us with energy, absorbing certain vitamins and minerals, and proper brain and nerve function. Although fats have a bad reputation, the right kinds of fats can actually be beneficial for our health.

The best food sources for fats

Fats are an essential part of any healthy diet and can be found in a wide variety of foods. Some of the best sources of fats include avocados, nuts, seeds, olives, fish, and fatty meats. Here is a closer look at each of these food sources and why they are beneficial.

Avocados: Avocados are a great source of healthy fats that can be beneficial to your health. Avocados are a type of fruit that contain monounsaturated fatty acids, which are known to help lower cholesterol levels and reduce the risk of heart disease. Additionally, avocados are a source of oleic acid, which has anti-inflammatory properties and can help protect against certain types of cancer. Avocados are also high in fibre and contain important vitamins, minerals, and antioxidants. They are an excellent source of potassium, which is important for maintaining healthy blood pressure and muscle health. Avocados are also high in vitamin K, which helps to promote healthy bones and blood clotting. Additionally, avocados provide magnesium, which is important for proper nerve and muscle function. Avocados are also high in healthy fats, containing about 14 grams of fat per one-third of an avocado. Most of the fats found in avocados are monounsaturated, which means they can help reduce your risk of heart disease. Monounsaturated fats are known to help lower bad cholesterol levels, while increasing good cholesterol levels. Additionally, monounsaturated fats can help reduce inflammation, which can benefit your overall health. Avocados also contain a variety of beneficial plant compounds, including carotenoids, polyphenols, and flavonoids, which can help protect against disease. One study found that avocados can help reduce the risk of certain types of cancer, such as prostate and breast cancer. Additionally, avocados can help protect against eye damage and reduce the risk of age-related macular degeneration. Overall, avocados are an excellent source of healthy fats that can provide many health benefits. Avocados are a great source of monounsaturated fats, which can help reduce cholesterol levels and reduce the risk of heart disease. Additionally, avocados are a great source of vitamins, minerals, and antioxidants that can help protect against disease. Avocados can be incorporated into a variety of meals or enjoyed as a snack, making them a great addition to any diet.

Nuts and Seeds: Nuts and seeds are an excellent source of healthy fats. They contain both monounsaturated and polyunsaturated fats, as well as essential fatty acids, which are essential for normal bodily functions. The fats found in nuts and seeds are also beneficial for heart health, as they can help reduce cholesterol levels and the risk of developing cardiovascular disease. Additionally, they are a great source of energy and can help keep you feeling full for longer, making them a great snack choice. Nuts and seeds are also a great source of protein, which is important for building and maintaining muscle. They are also rich in vitamins, minerals, and antioxidants that can help keep your body healthy. For example, they are high in magnesium, which is important for healthy bones and proper muscle function, and zinc, which is essential for a healthy immune system. Nuts and seeds are also a great source of fibre, which is important for a healthy digestive system. Eating a handful of nuts and seeds daily can help to keep your digestive system running smoothly and can help to reduce the risk of developing certain diseases. Finally, nuts and seeds are a great way to get your daily dose of healthy fats. Eating a handful of nuts and seeds every day can help to boost your overall health and may even help to reduce your risk of developing certain chronic diseases. So, if you're looking for a tasty and nutritious snack, look no further than nuts and seeds!

Olives: Olives are a great source of healthy fats, making them an essential part of a balanced diet. They contain monounsaturated fatty acids, which are beneficial for heart health and have been found to reduce cholesterol levels. Olives are also a great source of polyunsaturated fatty acids, which help to reduce inflammation and protect against chronic disease. The fatty acids in olives are beneficial for the body in many ways. They help promote the absorption of fat-soluble vitamins, such as Vitamin A, Vitamin D, and Vitamin E. They are also a great source of antioxidants, which help to protect cells from damage caused by free radicals. Additionally, olives contain oleic acid, which has been linked to a reduced risk of cancer. Olives are also a good source of fibre, which helps to keep the digestive system healthy and can help regulate blood sugar levels. Studies have also shown that the fatty acids in olives can help to reduce inflammation, which can be beneficial for those with arthritis or other inflammatory conditions. Overall, olives are a great source of healthy fats. They are packed with beneficial fatty acids, antioxidants, and fibre, which can all help to improve your health. They can be eaten as a snack, added to salads and other dishes, or used as an ingredient in cooking. Olives are a great addition to any diet and can help to provide essential nutrients and benefits to the body.

Fish: Fish is one of the best sources of dietary fats. Fats are an essential nutrient and provide a range of health benefits. They are required for normal growth and development and help to keep the body warm and provide energy. They also help to maintain healthy skin, hair and nails, and are necessary for the absorption of certain vitamins and minerals. Fish is a particularly good source of the so-called 'good' fats, namely omega-3 fatty acids. Omega-3 fatty acids are important for heart health and may help to reduce the risk of heart disease and stroke, as well as having beneficial effects on cholesterol levels and blood pressure. They can also help to reduce inflammation and may help to protect against some forms of cancer. Fish is also a great source of other beneficial fats, including monounsaturated and polyunsaturated fats. These fats are known to help improve cholesterol levels and reduce the risk of heart disease. They are also important for healthy brain development and may help to protect against mental decline. Fish is also a good source of other nutrients, including high-quality proteins, vitamins and minerals. Eating fish can help to increase intake of important nutrients such as calcium, zinc, selenium and iodine. In conclusion, fish is an excellent source of dietary fats. It is a good source of the 'good' fats, including omega-3 fatty acids, as well as other beneficial fats such as monounsaturated and polyunsaturated fats. Fish is also a good source of other important nutrients, including high-quality proteins, vitamins and minerals. Eating fish can help to improve overall health and reduce the risk of various diseases.

Fatty Meats: Fatty meats are an excellent source of dietary fats, providing a wide range of essential fatty acids and other important nutrients. Fatty meats are often high in monounsaturated fats, polyunsaturated fats, and saturated fats, all of which are important for maintaining good health. Monounsaturated fats are known to reduce levels of "bad" LDL cholesterol, while increasing levels of "good" HDL cholesterol. This type of fat is also associated with a reduced risk of heart disease, stroke, and diabetes. Polyunsaturated fats have similar benefits and are known to help reduce inflammation in the body and improve the health of the brain, heart, and other organs. Saturated fats are often vilified, but they actually have a number of health benefits. They provide the body with energy, help absorb fat-soluble vitamins, and are necessary for proper hormone production. Fatty meats are also a great source of protein and other important nutrients. Protein is critical for building and maintaining muscle mass and is essential for a healthy immune system. Fatty meats are also a good source of B vitamins, zinc, iron, and selenium. B vitamins help the body convert food into energy, while zinc and selenium are important for healthy immune function. Finally, fatty meats are a great way to get healthy omega-3 fatty acids. Omega-3s are essential fatty acids that cannot be produced by the body and must be obtained through diet. They are known to reduce inflammation, improve heart health, and protect against a number of chronic diseases. In conclusion, fatty meats are a great source of essential fatty acids and other important nutrients. They can help reduce levels of "bad" cholesterol, reduce inflammation, and provide the body with important vitamins and minerals.

For these reasons, fatty meats can be a healthy part of any diet.

Dairy: Diary products are an important part of a balanced diet and can provide a range of health benefits. They are a good source of essential fats, which are the building blocks for healthy cells and hormones. Fats from dairy provide essential fatty acids that can help to keep our skin, hair and nails healthy and strong. Dairy fats can also help to provide energy and support our metabolism. Dairy products are a great way to get the necessary fat for a healthy diet. Milk, cheese, yogurt and other dairy products are good sources of saturated and unsaturated fats. Saturated fats are found in high-fat dairy products like butter, cream and full-fat cheese, while unsaturated fats are found in lower-fat varieties like skimmed milk and low-fat cheese. In addition to providing essential fats, dairy products are also a good source of protein. Protein is essential for building and maintaining muscle and can help to keep us feeling fuller for longer. Dairy products are also packed with essential vitamins and minerals such as calcium, phosphorus, magnesium and vitamin D. These vitamins and minerals can help to keep our bones and teeth strong and support our immune system. Dairy products can also help to reduce the risk of developing certain chronic diseases. Studies have shown that consuming dairy products can reduce the risk of developing type 2 diabetes, heart disease and some forms of cancer. Dairy products are also a good source of probiotics, which can help to improve gut health. Overall, dairy products are a great way to get the essential fats, proteins, vitamins and minerals that our bodies need. They can provide a range of health benefits and help to reduce the risk of certain chronic diseases. For a balanced diet, it is important to include a variety of dairy products in your meals and snacks.

Dark chocolate: Dark chocolate is an excellent source of healthy fats, making it a great addition to a healthy diet. Not only are dark chocolates a good source of healthy fats, but they are also packed with antioxidants and minerals. The fats that are found in dark chocolate are mostly monounsaturated and polyunsaturated fats, which are known to be beneficial for heart health. These fats are also helpful in lowering cholesterol, reducing inflammation, and improving blood sugar levels. Dark chocolate also contains a lot of antioxidants, which can help protect the body from free radical damage. The antioxidants in dark chocolate can help reduce the risk of cancer and other chronic diseases. Dark chocolate is also a great source of magnesium, which is important for muscle and nerve function, and for maintaining healthy bones. Another benefit of dark chocolate is that it can help reduce cravings for unhealthy foods. Eating dark chocolate can help reduce cravings for sugar and other unhealthy snacks and can help you stay on track with your healthy eating habits. Finally, dark chocolate can be a great source of energy. Dark chocolate contains a small amount of caffeine, which can provide a boost of energy when you need it. It also contains theobromine, which is a natural stimulant that can help improve mood and focus. Overall, dark chocolate is an excellent source of healthy fats, antioxidants, and minerals. Eating dark chocolate can help reduce cravings for unhealthy snacks, provide a boost of energy, and improve overall health.

Why having too much is not good

Having too much fat in your diet can have serious consequences for your health. Eating too much fat can increase your risk of obesity, heart disease, stroke, and other chronic diseases. Excess fat can also lead to inflammation and other health problems. The main source of dietary fat is from animal-based foods such as meat, dairy, and eggs. Other sources of fat include oils, nuts, seeds, and avocados. Too much of these foods can increase your risk of developing health problems. Fats are important for the body to function properly, but too much fat can cause serious health problems. Eating too much saturated fat can raise cholesterol levels, which increases the risk of heart disease. Trans fats, which are found in processed foods, can also raise cholesterol levels and increase the risk of heart disease. Eating too much fat can also lead to weight gain. Fats are more calorie-dense than other nutrients, so eating a lot of fatty foods can cause you to consume too many calories. This can lead to weight gain, which in turn increases the risk of other health problems. Excess fat can also lead to inflammation. The body needs a certain amount of fat to function properly, but too much fat can cause inflammation, which can lead to a range of health problems, including joint pain, diabetes, and cancer. Finally, eating too much fat can also have an effect on your mental health. Eating a diet high in fat can cause mood swings, depression, and anxiety. Overall, it's important to maintain a healthy balance of fats in your diet. Eating too much fat can increase your risk of obesity, heart disease, stroke, and other chronic diseases. It's important to choose healthy fats, such as olive oil, nuts, and avocados, and limit your intake of saturated and trans fats.

Eating a variety of these foods can help you get the fat you need for good health. However, it's important to remember that all fats should be consumed in moderation. Too much fat can lead to weight gain and increase the risk of health problems.

MINERALS

Minerals are naturally occurring substances, formed over time by geological processes. They are essential for life and form the basis of our environment. They can be found in rocks, soil, water, and air. They are classified into two main groups: organic and inorganic. Organic minerals are those that are made up of elements that were once living organisms, such as carbon, nitrogen, and phosphorus. These minerals are important for the growth and development of plants and animals. Examples include calcium, phosphorus, and magnesium. Inorganic minerals are those that are formed without the influence of organisms. They are formed through chemical and physical processes, such as volcanic eruptions, weathering, and erosion. Examples include iron, aluminium, and sodium. Minerals are found in abundance in the Earth's crust and are a major component of rocks and soils. They can also be found in sedimentary rocks, such as limestone, and in groundwater. Minerals are essential for life as they provide the body with essential nutrients, such as calcium and phosphorus, which are necessary for the growth and repair of bones and teeth. They are also necessary for the formation of hormones, enzymes, and other compounds necessary for normal body functions.

Minerals are essential for human health and development. They provide many of the body's functions and are needed for growth and development. Minerals play an important role in many body functions, from forming bones to regulating muscle contractions, from regulating fluid balance to delivering oxygen to cells. Minerals are also important for maintaining healthy skin, hair, and nails. The most important minerals for the human body are calcium, phosphorus, magnesium, iron, potassium, sodium, zinc, and selenium. Calcium is needed for strong bones and teeth, as well as nerve and muscle function. Phosphorus helps the body use carbohydrates, protein, and fat, as well as maintain a healthy acid-base balance. Magnesium is important for energy production, muscle and nerve function, and regulating blood sugar levels. Iron is needed to make haemoglobin, which is responsible for carrying oxygen in the blood. Potassium helps regulate the water balance and muscle contractions. Sodium helps regulate blood pressure and nerve impulses. Zinc is needed for growth and development, tissue repair, and the immune system. Selenium helps protect cells from damage and is essential for proper thyroid function. Minerals are found in a variety of foods, including fruits, vegetables, meats, fish, nuts, and grains. Foods that are rich in minerals include dark, leafy greens, legumes, nuts, seeds, fortified cereals and grains, and dairy products. Eating a balanced diet that is rich in minerals can help ensure that you get the nutrients you need to stay healthy. Getting enough minerals from your diet is important for overall health and well-being. Minerals are essential for maintaining strong bones, healthy teeth, and proper muscle and nerve function. They play a role in energy production, cell growth, and regulating hormones. Minerals are also important for maintaining a healthy immune system and protecting cells from damage. By eating a variety of foods that are rich in minerals, you can ensure that you are getting the nutrients you need to stay healthy.

Calcium

Calcium is an essential mineral that plays a vital role in many body functions, including nerve transmission, muscle contraction, and blood clotting. It is one of the most abundant minerals in the human body, and it is found in many foods, such as dairy products, green leafy vegetables, and certain fish. Calcium is necessary for building and maintaining strong bones and teeth, and it is important for the proper functioning of the heart, muscles, and nerves. It also helps regulate blood pressure and clotting, and it is important for a healthy immune system. Calcium is absorbed by the body in the small intestine and is then transported to the bones and teeth, where it is stored for later use. It is also released into the bloodstream to help regulate muscle contraction, nerve transmission, and blood clotting. Calcium is found in many foods, including dairy products such as milk, cheese, and yogurt; fortified cereals; green leafy vegetables such as spinach and kale; and certain fish such as salmon and sardines. Calcium supplements are also available and may be recommended by a doctor if dietary sources of calcium are insufficient. It is important to note that calcium is best absorbed when it is consumed with food and that it is important to get enough vitamin D to help the body absorb calcium. Vitamin D is found in foods such as eggs, fatty fish, and fortified milk, as well as in supplements. Getting adequate amounts of calcium is important for overall health, and it is especially important for children and teenagers, who are still growing and need a steady supply of calcium for their bones and teeth. It is also important for pregnant and breastfeeding women to ensure they are getting enough calcium in their diets. Calcium is an essential mineral that plays a vital role in many body functions, and it is important for overall health. It is found in many foods, including dairy products, green leafy vegetables, and certain fish, and supplements are available if dietary sources are insufficient. Getting enough calcium is especially important for children, teenagers, pregnant women, and breastfeeding women.

Calcium is an essential nutrient for strong bones and teeth, muscle and nerve function, and hormone production. It also helps to regulate blood pressure, maintain normal heartbeat, and helps the body absorb and use other essential nutrients. Calcium helps to keep bones and teeth strong by providing the building blocks for the body to produce bones. Calcium helps to create a strong skeletal system, which helps protect the body from injury and deformity. Calcium also helps to regulate the contraction and relaxation of muscles, including those of the heart, which is important for a healthy cardiovascular system. Calcium is also important for the functioning of the nervous system. It helps to transmit nerve impulses, allowing the body to coordinate movement and sensation. Calcium also helps to regulate hormone production, which affects metabolism, reproduction, and stress responses. In addition to its many important functions in the body, calcium is also important for overall health. A lack of calcium can lead to a number of health issues, including osteoporosis, tooth decay, and even an increased risk of certain types of cancer. Calcium also plays an important role in preventing or delaying the onset of age-related conditions, such as Alzheimer's disease. Adults should aim to consume at least 1000-1300 mg of calcium each day. Good sources of calcium include dairy products, such as milk, yogurt, and cheese, as well as certain types of fish, nuts, and green leafy vegetables. Certain types of fortified cereals and juices can also provide a good source of calcium. Supplements can also be taken to help meet daily calcium needs. Overall, calcium is an essential mineral for the human body, playing a crucial role in many of its functions. It is important for strong bones and teeth, muscle and nerve function, and hormone production, and helps to regulate blood pressure and maintain normal heartbeat. For adults, it is recommended to get at least 1000-1300 mg of calcium each day, from dietary sources or supplements.

The Best Food Sources for Calcium

Calcium is a very important mineral for our body, as it is essential for healthy bones and teeth, as well as for proper muscle and nerve functioning. It is also important for maintaining a healthy circulatory system. While dairy products are often thought of as the best sources of calcium, there are many other sources of this essential mineral. Here are some of the best food sources for calcium:

Dairy Products: Calcium is an essential mineral found in dairy products, such as milk, yogurt, and cheese. It plays a vital role in maintaining strong bones and teeth, as well as helping with nerve and muscle function. Calcium is also important for blood clotting and maintaining a healthy heart. Dairy products are the best source of calcium. Milk, yogurt, and cheese are especially rich in calcium, providing around 300 mg per 8-ounce serving. Other dairy products, such as cottage cheese and ice cream, also contain calcium, though in smaller amounts. Calcium is important for bone health. It helps form new bone and keeps bones strong and healthy. It also helps with muscle contraction and nerve transmission. For these reasons, it's important to get enough calcium in your diet. Adults need about 1000 mg of calcium a day. It's recommended that adults get three servings of dairy per day to meet this requirement. This could be in the form of 8-ounce glasses of milk, 8-ounce containers of yogurt, or 1.5 ounces of cheese. For those who can't or don't consume dairy, there are other ways to get calcium. Some non-dairy sources of calcium include dark leafy greens, such as kale and spinach, and calcium-fortified foods, such as soy milk and orange juice. It's worth noting that calcium is best absorbed when taken with vitamin D, so it's important to get enough of both in your diet. Vitamin D can be found in fortified dairy products, egg yolks, fatty fish, and some mushrooms. In conclusion, dairy products are an excellent source of calcium, and they're essential for maintaining strong bones and teeth. Adults should aim to get three servings of dairy per day to meet their calcium requirements. For those who don't or can't consume dairy, there are other sources of calcium, including dark leafy greens and calcium-fortified products.

Green Leafy Vegetables: . Calcium is an essential mineral that plays a vital role in many bodily functions, particularly bone health. Leafy greens are one of the best sources of calcium, providing a range of benefits to our health. Leafy greens are a type of vegetable that includes spinach, kale, collard greens, and Swiss chard. These vegetables are packed with essential vitamins, minerals, and antioxidants. Calcium is one of these essential minerals, and it is found in high concentrations in leafy greens. Calcium is an important mineral for our bodies, and it has many benefits. It helps to build and maintain strong bones, it is essential for nerve and muscle function, and it helps to regulate the acid-base balance in our blood. Calcium is also important for blood clotting, hormone regulation, and metabolism. Consuming calcium-rich foods such as leafy greens is important for maintaining healthy bones and teeth and for reducing the risk of osteoporosis. Leafy greens contain more calcium than other vegetables, such as broccoli and cauliflower. A single cup of cooked spinach contains over 250 milligrams of calcium, which is 25% of the recommended daily intake for adults. Other leafy greens such as kale, collard greens, and Swiss chard also provide significant amounts of calcium. In addition to providing calcium, leafy greens are also loaded with other essential vitamins and minerals. These include vitamins A, C, and K, as well as potassium, magnesium, and iron. The antioxidants found in leafy greens also help to protect our cells from damage. Eating leafy greens is a simple and delicious way to get your daily dose of calcium. Leafy greens can be eaten raw or cooked, and can be added to salads, soups, stir-fries, and smoothies. Leafy greens are also low in calories and high in fibre, making them a nutritious addition to any meal. In conclusion, leafy greens are an excellent source of calcium and other essential vitamins and minerals. Eating leafy greens can help to keep your bones and teeth strong, reduce your risk of osteoporosis, and provide other health benefits. Make sure to include leafy greens in your diet for optimal health.

Fish: Calcium is an essential mineral for every living organism and fish are no exception. It is essential for the development and maintenance of strong bones, healthy teeth, and normal muscle function. Calcium is found in a variety of fish in different concentrations, depending on the species. It can also be obtained from other sources such as algae and other aquatic plants. Calcium is necessary for many of the physiological processes in fish. It plays a role in the development of strong bones, maintaining healthy teeth, and normal muscle function. Calcium is also important for several biochemical processes, including blood clotting, nerve transmission, and enzyme function. In addition, calcium helps regulate the metabolism in fish. The concentration of calcium in fish varies depending on the species. For example, some species, such as salmon, contain higher levels of calcium than others, such as mackerel. The level of calcium in fish also depends on the water they live in. For example, fish that live in hard water are likely to have higher levels of calcium compared to those that live in soft water. It is important to ensure that fish have an adequate supply of calcium to stay healthy. There are several ways to do this, such as providing a balanced diet containing the right mix of fish food and supplements. Many fish foods contain calcium in the form of calcium carbonate or calcium gluconate. Supplements can also be added to the water or added directly to the fish food. In summary, calcium is an essential mineral for fish. It is necessary for the development and maintenance of strong bones, healthy teeth, and normal muscle function. The concentration of calcium in fish varies depending on the species and can be obtained from other sources such as algae and other aquatic plants. It is important to ensure that fish have an adequate supply of calcium to stay healthy by providing a balanced diet of fish food and supplements.

Fortified Cereals and Grains: Calcium is an essential mineral for a healthy body. It is necessary for strong bones, healthy muscles and normal nerve functioning. Unfortunately, many people don't get enough calcium in their diet. This is why many foods, including fortified cereals and grains, are now fortified with calcium. Fortified cereals and grains are foods that have had calcium added to them. This can be done in a variety of ways, but most commonly it involves adding calcium carbonate or calcium phosphate to the food. These calcium compounds are a form of calcium that is easy for the body to absorb and use. By adding these compounds to cereals and grains, manufacturers are able to provide a source of calcium that is readily available to the body. The amount of calcium added to cereals and grains varies depending on the product. Generally, fortified cereals and grains will have more calcium than non-fortified varieties. This means that people who are looking for a good source of calcium can benefit from choosing fortified products. In addition to providing a source of calcium, fortified cereals and grains also provide other key nutrients. For example, many fortified cereals and grains are also fortified with vitamins and minerals such as iron, magnesium and zinc. These vitamins and minerals are necessary for healthy bodily functions. By adding these to the food, manufacturers are able to provide an excellent source of nutrition. Overall, fortified cereals and grains are an excellent way to get the calcium you need. By choosing fortified products, you can ensure that you are getting enough of this essential mineral. Additionally, you can benefit from the other key nutrients that are included in fortified products. If you are looking for a good source of calcium, fortified cereals and grains are a great choice.

Nuts and Seeds: Nuts are a great source of calcium, as they are packed full of nutrients and minerals. Almonds are one of the best sources, providing an impressive 75mg of calcium in just one ounce. Walnuts are also a great source, containing 25mg of calcium per ounce. Other nuts such as cashews, hazelnuts, macadamias and pecans all contain significant amounts of calcium too. Seeds are also an excellent source of calcium, containing around 7-20mg per tablespoon, depending on the type of seed. Sesame seeds are one of the best sources, providing 35mg of calcium in just one tablespoon. Other seeds such as sunflower, flax and pumpkin all contain significant amounts of calcium too. Nuts and seeds are also great sources of other minerals and vitamins too. Almonds, for example, are a great source of vitamin E, which helps to protect cells from damage and can also help to reduce inflammation in the body. Walnuts are a great source of omega-3 fatty acids, which are essential for a healthy heart. Flax seeds are a great source of fibre and are also a good source of magnesium, which helps to regulate blood sugar levels. Nuts and seeds are an incredibly versatile food source and can be added to a variety of dishes, from salads to smoothies. They can also be eaten on their own as a healthy snack. Eating nuts and seeds regularly is a great way to boost your calcium intake and ensure that you are getting the essential nutrients that your body needs.

Legumes: While dairy products are a widely known source of this mineral, legumes are also a great source of calcium. Legumes are a type of plant that produces seeds inside a pod, such as beans, peanuts, and peas. Legumes contain high amounts of calcium, with some types containing up to 200 milligrams per serving. This amount is equivalent to about 20% of the daily recommended intake for adults. Soybeans, in particular, contain particularly high levels of calcium, with some varieties offering up to 250 milligrams per serving. Legumes are also a good source of other essential minerals like iron, magnesium, zinc, and phosphorus. These minerals support bone health, muscle function, and other bodily processes. They also contain vitamins, such as vitamin K and folate, which are necessary for blood clotting and cell health, respectively. The calcium found in legumes is more easily absorbed than other plant sources, such as spinach. This means that the body can use the calcium more effectively. Additionally, legumes are a good source of dietary fibre, which helps to keep the digestive system functioning properly. Because legumes are a plant-based source of calcium, they may be a good choice for people who are lactose intolerant or vegan. They are also low in calories and fat, making them a healthy choice for those trying to lose weight. Legumes can be enjoyed in a variety of ways. They can be added to soups, salads, stews, stir-fries, and more. They can also be enjoyed as a snack or as a meal replacement. In summary, legumes are a great source of calcium and other essential minerals. They are more easily absorbed than other plant sources, making them a great choice for those who are lactose intolerant or vegan. They are also low in calories and fat, making them a healthy choice for those trying to lose weight. Legumes can be enjoyed in many different ways and should be included in a well-balanced diet.

Fruits: There are many fruits that provide an excellent source of this essential nutrient. Fruits that are high in calcium can make it easier to meet the daily recommended intake, which is 1,000 milligrams for adults and 1,300 milligrams for teenagers and adolescents. Oranges are one of the best sources of calcium. A single medium-sized orange can provide up to 80 milligrams of calcium, which is nearly 10% of the daily recommended intake. Oranges are also rich in vitamin C and antioxidants, which makes them a great choice for snacks or meals. Figs are another excellent source of calcium. A single cup of dried figs can provide up to 300 milligrams of calcium, which is more than 20% of the daily recommended intake. They are also high in fibre, potassium, and magnesium, making them a great choice for a healthy snack or meal. Kiwis are a great source of calcium, as well. A single kiwi can provide up to 30 milligrams of calcium, which is almost 4% of the daily recommended intake. Kiwis are also high in vitamin C and antioxidants, making them a great choice for a healthy snack or meal. Bananas are another great source of calcium. A single banana can provide up to 10 milligrams of calcium, which is 1% of the daily recommended intake. Bananas are also high in fibre and potassium, making them a great choice for a healthy snack or meal. Fruits are a great way to get more calcium into your diet. Not only do they provide essential nutrients, but they are also a delicious and convenient way to get your daily recommended intake of calcium. Eating a variety of fruits that are high in calcium can help you reach your daily calcium goals and keep your bones and teeth strong and healthy.

Adding dairy products, green leafy vegetables, fish, fortified cereals and grains, nuts and seeds, legumes, and fruits to your diet is a great way to get enough calcium and other essential nutrients.

Potassium

Potassium is a mineral and an electrolyte that is essential to life, and which helps to regulate the body's fluid balance. It plays an important role in regulating blood pressure and the body's pH levels, as well as helping to transmit nerve signals. It is also necessary for muscle contraction and the production of energy. Potassium is found in many foods, including fruit, vegetables, legumes, dairy, fish, and meat. It is also added to some processed foods as a preservative. The body cannot produce potassium on its own and gets most of it from dietary sources. The daily recommended intake of potassium is 4,700 milligrams, although this can vary depending on age, sex, and other health factors. Potassium is involved in a number of processes in the body, including nerve transmission, muscle contraction, and the production of energy. It helps to regulate blood pressure and the body's pH balance by maintaining the optimal balance of sodium and potassium in the blood. It also helps to maintain the body's fluid balance and the electrolyte balance, which is important for proper functioning of the cells. Potassium deficiency can lead to a number of symptoms, including muscle weakness, fatigue, and difficulty concentrating. In extreme cases, it can lead to an irregular heartbeat or even a heart attack. Too much potassium can also be dangerous, leading to a condition known as hyperkalaemia, which can cause kidney failure, paralysis, and even death. For most people, a balanced diet should provide enough potassium. If you are at risk of developing a potassium imbalance, or if you have a medical condition that affects your ability to absorb potassium, your doctor may recommend that you take potassium supplements or eat more potassium-rich foods.

Potassium is an essential mineral that plays an important

role in maintaining good health. It is required for a variety of bodily functions, including regulating the balance of fluids and electrolytes in the body, assisting in muscle contraction, and helping to maintain normal nerve and heart function. Potassium is also important for bone health, as it helps to regulate calcium and phosphorus levels. The recommended daily intake of potassium for adults is 4,700 milligrams per day. This can be obtained from a variety of sources, including fruits, vegetables, legumes and dairy products. Eating foods that are high in potassium can help to ensure that the body is getting enough of the mineral. One of the main benefits of potassium is that it helps to regulate the amount of sodium in the body. Sodium is an electrolyte that can cause high blood pressure when consumed in excess. Potassium helps to balance out the effects of sodium in the body, helping to maintain a healthy blood pressure. Potassium is also important for muscle health. It helps to regulate muscle contraction, which is essential for physical activity. It also helps to maintain normal nerve and heart function, which is essential for overall health. Potassium is also important for bone health, as it helps to regulate calcium and phosphorus levels. Calcium and phosphorus are two essential minerals that are needed for strong and healthy bones. Without adequate levels of these minerals, bones can become weak and brittle. In addition, potassium is important for maintaining healthy blood sugar levels. Studies have shown that a high-potassium diet can help to lower blood sugar levels in individuals with type 2 diabetes. Finally, potassium can help to reduce the risk of stroke. Studies have shown that individuals who consume higher amounts of potassium have a lower risk of stroke than those who consume lower amounts. In summary, potassium is an important mineral for overall health, and consuming enough of it can help to ensure that the body is functioning optimally. Eating a diet that is high in fruits, vegetables, legumes and dairy products is the best way to ensure that the body is getting enough of the mineral.

Food sources

Potassium is an essential mineral that plays an important role in the body's health. It helps to regulate blood pressure, electrolyte balance, and muscle contraction. It is also necessary for the proper functioning of the heart, kidneys, and other organs. A diet that is rich in potassium can help to reduce the risk of stroke, high blood pressure, and other health conditions. The best food sources for potassium are fruits, vegetables, beans, and dairy products.

Bananas: Bananas are one of the most widely consumed fruits in the world and are a great source of nutrition. They are also rich in many essential vitamins and minerals, including potassium. Potassium is an essential mineral that helps to regulate the body's fluid balance, nerve function, and heart rate. It also helps to maintain healthy blood pressure levels and can help to reduce the risk of stroke and heart disease. Bananas are an excellent source of dietary potassium. One medium-sized banana contains 422 milligrams of potassium, or about 10% of the daily recommended value. Bananas are also relatively low in calories and contain no cholesterol or fat. Bananas are a great source of dietary fibre and provide essential vitamins and minerals. In addition to potassium, bananas are also a good source of vitamin B6, vitamin C, manganese, and magnesium. They are also a good source of dietary fibre, which can help to lower cholesterol levels and aid digestion. Bananas are a convenient and healthy snack and can be eaten on their own or added to smoothies and other recipes. They are also an excellent addition to breakfast cereals and can be used as an ingredient in baking. Bananas can also be frozen and used in smoothies or as an ice cream topping. In conclusion, bananas are a nutritious and convenient snack that are packed with essential vitamins and minerals. They are an excellent source of dietary potassium, which is essential for healthy blood pressure levels and nerve and muscle function. Bananas can be eaten on their own or added to a variety of recipes to boost their nutritional value.

Oranges: Oranges are a popular citrus fruit, and a great source of nutrition for many people. They are full of a variety of vitamins and minerals, including potassium. Oranges are one of the best sources of potassium, providing about 10% of the recommended daily amount in just one small orange. Eating one orange a day can help to ensure adequate levels of this essential mineral in the body. This is especially important for people who may not be getting enough potassium from their diet. Oranges are also a great source of other vitamins and minerals, including vitamin C, fibre, magnesium, and calcium. They are a good source of antioxidants and can help to reduce inflammation in the body. Eating oranges regularly can also help to boost the immune system and reduce the risk of certain diseases. Overall, oranges are an excellent source of potassium, as well as other essential vitamins and minerals. Eating oranges regularly can help to ensure adequate levels of this essential mineral in the body, as well as providing other health benefits. So, if you're looking for a delicious and nutritious way to get your daily dose of potassium, adding more oranges to your diet is a great way to do it.

Grapefruit: Grapefruit is a citrus fruit that is known for its tangy and sweet taste. It is packed with essential vitamins and minerals, but one of the most notable nutrients found in grapefruit is potassium. A single medium-sized grapefruit contains about 274 milligrams of potassium. This is equivalent to about 8% of the recommended daily intake for adults. Potassium is known for its ability to help regulate blood pressure. The mineral helps to reduce the amount of sodium in the body, which can help to lower blood pressure. Studies have shown that a diet high in potassium can help to reduce the risk of stroke and other cardiovascular diseases. Potassium is also important for muscle function. The mineral helps to maintain fluid balance in the body, which can help to reduce muscle cramps and fatigue. It can also help to reduce the risk of muscle weakness and help to build muscle mass. Grapefruit is a great source of potassium, but it is important to note that it can interact with certain medications. Grapefruit juice can interact with some medications, and it is important to speak to your doctor before consuming grapefruit or grapefruit juice if you are taking any medications. Overall, grapefruit is an excellent source of potassium. It can help to regulate blood pressure, support heart health, and maintain muscle function. However, it is important to speak to your doctor before consuming grapefruit or grapefruit juice if you are taking any medications.

Kiwi: Kiwi is a nutrient-rich fruit packed with essential vitamins, minerals, and antioxidants. One of the most beneficial minerals found in kiwi is potassium, which is an essential electrolyte necessary for the proper functioning of the body. Kiwi is an excellent source of potassium. Just one medium kiwi contains about 250 mg of potassium, which is nearly 6 percent of the daily recommended value. This makes kiwi a great food for people looking to increase their potassium intake. Kiwi is also a good source of dietary fibre and vitamin C. Dietary fibre helps to support good digestive health and vitamin C is important for immune health and collagen synthesis. In addition to its many health benefits, kiwi is also low in calories and fat, making it a great snack for those looking to lose weight. In summary, kiwi is a nutrient-rich fruit packed with essential minerals, vitamins, and antioxidants. Of these, potassium is an important electrolyte necessary for the body's proper functioning. Kiwi is an excellent source of potassium, providing nearly 6 percent of the daily recommended value in just one medium kiwi. In addition to its potassium content, kiwi is also a good source of dietary fibre and vitamin C, making it a great snack for those looking to lose weight.

Broccoli: Potassium is an essential mineral that can be found in many vegetables, including broccoli. Broccoli is an especially good source of potassium, providing more than 200 milligrams per cup. This amount is more than 10 percent of the daily recommended intake for adults. Potassium is important for the body in many ways. It helps regulate fluid balance, muscle contractions, and nerve signals. It also helps to reduce the risk of stroke, high blood pressure, heart disease, and kidney stones. Potassium is found in both the stems and florets of broccoli, with the highest concentration being in the florets. One cup of cooked broccoli contains about 220 milligrams of potassium. This amount is almost the same as one banana, though the potassium in broccoli is less readily absorbed into the body than in a banana. In addition to providing potassium, broccoli is also a great source of other important vitamins and minerals. It is high in vitamins C, K, and A, as well as folate and fibre. It also contains calcium, magnesium, phosphorus, and iron. The health benefits of broccoli are further enhanced when it is eaten raw or lightly steamed. This allows the vegetable to retain more of its nutrients, including potassium. Overall, broccoli is an excellent source of potassium, as well as many other important vitamins and minerals. Eating it regularly can help to maintain healthy blood pressure, reduce the risk of stroke and heart disease, and keep bones strong and healthy.

Spinach: Potassium is an essential mineral that is found in many vegetables, including spinach. It is an electrolyte, which means it helps to regulate the electrical activity in the body. Potassium helps to regulate fluid balance, nerve signals, and muscle contractions. It also helps to keep the heart beating regularly and may help to lower blood pressure. Spinach is a great source of potassium. A cup of cooked spinach contains 839 milligrams of potassium, which is 20% of the recommended daily intake of 4,700 milligrams. Eating a diet that is rich in potassium can help to reduce the risk of stroke, heart disease, and kidney stones. It may also help to reduce the risk of developing type 2 diabetes. Potassium is important for muscle strength and contraction. It helps to send nerve signals to the muscles, which allows them to move. Eating a diet that is rich in potassium can help to reduce muscle cramps and fatigue. It may also help to improve strength and endurance during exercise. Potassium is also important for bone health. It helps to keep bones strong and healthy by regulating calcium levels in the body. Spinach is also a good source of other minerals, such as magnesium and calcium, which are important for bone health. Potassium is important for maintaining healthy blood pressure. Eating a diet that is rich in potassium can help to reduce the risk of high blood pressure and stroke. Spinach is also a good source of dietary fibre, which can help to reduce cholesterol levels. In conclusion, spinach is a great source of potassium. Eating a diet that is rich in potassium can help to keep the heart healthy, reduce the risk of stroke, and improve muscle strength and endurance. Spinach is also a good source of other minerals, such as magnesium and calcium, which are important for bone health. Eating a diet that is rich in potassium can also help to reduce the risk of high blood pressure and stroke.

Potatoes: Potatoes are one of the most popular vegetables around the world. They are a good source of nutrients, including potassium. Potassium is a mineral that is essential for the proper functioning of the body's cells, tissues, and organs. It helps regulate blood pressure and heart rate, maintains fluid balance, and helps the body make proteins and break down carbohydrates. One medium-size potato (about 5.3 ounces) contains 620 milligrams (mg) of potassium, which is about 13 percent of the recommended daily value. Potatoes also contain other minerals, including magnesium and phosphorus. It is also important for nerve and muscle function and helps the body absorb calcium, which is essential for strong bones and teeth. Eating foods that are rich in potassium can help lower blood pressure and reduce the risk of stroke, heart attack, and other cardiovascular diseases. Potassium can also help prevent kidney stones and reduce the risk of osteoporosis. Some people may be at risk for developing a potassium deficiency. This can be caused by certain medications, chronic kidney disease, or excessive sweating. Symptoms of a potassium deficiency include fatigue, muscle weakness, and irregular heartbeat. Eating a balanced diet that includes potatoes and other potassium-rich foods can help ensure adequate intake and reduce the risk of deficiency. Potatoes are also a good source of fibre, vitamin C, and other vitamins and minerals. Eating a variety of fruits and vegetables every day can help ensure that you get all the nutrients you need.

Tomatoes: Potassium is an essential nutrient for humans and is found in many foods, including tomatoes. Tomatoes are a great source of potassium, with one medium-sized tomato providing about 294 milligrams of the mineral. This amount is about 8 percent of the daily recommended intake for an adult. Tomatoes are also a good source of other essential nutrients, such as vitamin C, vitamin A, and fibre. They also contain lycopene, an antioxidant that has been found to have a number of health benefits, including reducing the risk of some types of cancer. When buying tomatoes, it is important to look for those that are ripe, as they will contain the highest amounts of potassium. It is also important to store tomatoes correctly, as they can lose some of their nutritional value when exposed to light or heat. Tomatoes can be enjoyed in a variety of ways. They can be eaten raw, in salads, or cooked in sauces, soups, and other dishes. They can also be used to make sauces, salsas, and other condiments. Tomatoes are an easy way to increase the amount of potassium in your diet and get the health benefits associated with it.

Kidney Beans: Potassium is an essential mineral nutrient found in many foods, and kidney beans are no exception. Kidney beans are a great source of dietary potassium. One cup of cooked kidney beans contains about 600 milligrams of potassium, which is about 15 percent of the recommended daily intake. This amount is enough to meet the needs of most adults, including pregnant and breastfeeding women. Kidney beans are an excellent source of dietary potassium, providing more than half of the recommended daily intake in one cup. Kidney beans are also a great source of other vitamins and minerals, including iron, magnesium, and zinc. They are low in fat and calories and high in fibre, making them a nutritious addition to any diet. In addition to providing dietary potassium, kidney beans are also rich in phytonutrients, which are plant compounds that have antioxidant and anti-inflammatory properties. Phytonutrients have been linked to a number of health benefits, including a reduced risk of cancer and heart disease. Overall, kidney beans are an excellent source of dietary potassium, as well as other essential vitamins and minerals. Eating a diet rich in potassium-rich foods can help reduce the risk of developing high blood pressure, stroke, and heart disease, and may also help protect against certain types of cancer. Incorporating kidney beans into your diet can be an easy way to get the potassium and other nutrients your body needs.

Pinto Beans: Pinto beans are a type of legume, and they are a popular source of nutrition in many cultures. They are packed with protein, vitamins, minerals, and other essential nutrients. One of the key minerals found in pinto beans is potassium. Potassium is a mineral essential for the proper functioning of the human body. It helps to regulate muscle contractions, including the heartbeat, and it is important for maintaining a healthy balance of fluids. It is also necessary for proper nerve conduction and for the efficient absorption of glucose. Pinto beans are an excellent source of potassium. One cup of cooked pinto beans provides around 564 milligrams of potassium, which is about 16 percent of the recommended daily intake for adults. This amount of potassium is equivalent to what is found in one medium banana. Potassium also helps to regulate electrolyte balance, which helps to prevent dehydration. In addition to potassium, pinto beans are also a great source of fibre, protein, and other essential vitamins and minerals. Pinto beans are also low in fat and sodium, making them a healthy choice for those looking to reduce their intake of unhealthy fats and sodium. Pinto beans can be enjoyed in a variety of dishes, from soups and stews to salads and burritos. They can also be mashed and used as a spread on toast or crackers. Pinto beans can also be used in place of ground beef in dishes like tacos and chili. In conclusion, pinto beans are an excellent source of potassium and other essential nutrients. They are low in fat and sodium, and they can be enjoyed in a variety of dishes. Eating pinto beans can help to reduce the risk of stroke and coronary heart disease, and it can also help to maintain a healthy balance of fluids in the body.

Black Beans: Potassium is found in a variety of foods, including black beans. Black beans are a delicious, nutritious legume that is often used in a variety of dishes, from salads to soups. They are also an excellent source of plant-based protein, fibre, and minerals like potassium. One cup of cooked black beans contains about 740 mg of potassium. This amount is roughly 20 percent of the recommended daily intake for adults. Potassium helps regulate the balance of fluids in the body and helps move nutrients into cells. It also plays a role in muscle contractions, nerve transmission, and heart health. Research has suggested that getting enough potassium in your diet can help decrease the risk of stroke, kidney stones, and osteoporosis. Potassium is lost during the cooking process, so it is important to use a low-sodium cooking method when preparing black beans. To reduce sodium, rinse the beans before cooking them and use water instead of broth or stock. Adding potassium-rich foods to the cooking liquid, like tomatoes or potatoes, can also help increase the amount of potassium in your meal. In addition to providing potassium, black beans are also a good source of protein, dietary fibre, iron, magnesium, and folate. They are low in fat and have no cholesterol, making them an excellent choice for people looking to reduce their risk of heart disease. Eating black beans can also help you feel fuller for longer, making them a great choice for weight loss. Eating black beans regularly can be an easy way to get more potassium into your diet. They are also a delicious and nutritious addition to many meals. Try adding them to salads, soups, stews, and casseroles for a nutritious and flavourful boost of potassium.

Milk: Milk is a great source of potassium, as it contains roughly 160 milligrams per cup. This is approximately 5% of the recommended daily intake of the mineral. It is also relatively easily absorbed by the body, making it a great way to get your daily dose. In order to get the most out of the potassium found in milk, it is important to choose low-fat or fat-free varieties. These still contain the same amount of potassium, but without the added calories. It is also important to drink plenty of water, as this will help to flush the potassium out of the body. Overall, potassium is an essential mineral that is found in many foods, including milk. It is important for a number of reasons, including maintaining fluid balance and reducing the risk of stroke and heart disease. It is also essential for those trying to lose weight, as it can help to reduce the bloating caused by too much sodium. For those looking to get the most out of the potassium found in milk, it is important to choose low-fat or fat-free varieties, and to drink plenty of water.

Yogurt: Yogurt is a popular snack and breakfast food that is packed with nutrients. One of the essential nutrients that yogurt provides is potassium. Potassium is a mineral that is essential for maintaining healthy blood pressure and heart function. It is also important for nerve and muscle function, as well as for building strong bones. When it comes to yogurt, there are many varieties and flavours available on the market. But not all yogurts are created equal when it comes to their potassium content. Plain non-fat yogurt is generally the best source of potassium, as it contains the most potassium per serving. One cup of plain non-fat yogurt can contain up to 534 milligrams of potassium, which is about 15% of your daily recommended value. Yogurt can also be a great source of other essential nutrients, such as protein and calcium. Greek yogurt, in particular, is a great source of protein as it contains twice the amount of protein than regular yogurt. It also contains more calcium than regular yogurt, which is important for bone health. If you are looking for a snack that is high in potassium, yogurt can be a great choice. But it is important to remember that not all yogurts are created equal, and some varieties can contain added sugar and other unhealthy ingredients. To ensure you are getting the most health benefits from your yogurt, it is best to opt for plain, non-fat yogurt whenever possible. Additionally, you can top your yogurt with fruit, nuts, or other nutritious toppings to add a boost of flavour while also increasing its nutritional value.

Cheese: Cheese is an incredibly popular food, whether it is used in dishes or simply eaten on its own. It is known for its rich flavour and creamy texture, but it is also packed with nutrients. One of the most important nutrients found in cheese is potassium. The amount of potassium in cheese depends on the type of cheese. For instance, cheddar cheese contains a higher amount of potassium than Swiss cheese. In general, a one ounce serving of cheese contains between 150 and 200 milligrams of potassium. This is equivalent to 4 to 5% of the recommended daily value. In addition to providing an excellent source of potassium, cheese is also a good source of other nutrients, such as calcium, phosphorus, and magnesium. These minerals help to maintain healthy bones, teeth, and muscles. Cheese also contains a variety of vitamins, such as B vitamins, vitamin A, and vitamin D. Overall, cheese is an excellent food to include in your diet because it is packed with nutrients that are important for your health. The potassium in cheese is particularly beneficial because it helps to regulate blood pressure, heart rate, and water balance in the body. In addition, cheese is a good source of other minerals and vitamins that are important for maintaining healthy bones, teeth, and muscles.

Phosphorus

Phosphorus is an essential mineral that plays a key role in the body's growth, development and maintenance of healthy bones and teeth. It is found in all living organisms, including plants and animals. Phosphorus is also important to many metabolic processes and helps to convert food into energy. In food, phosphorus can be found in a variety of sources, such as dairy products, eggs, fish, poultry, legumes, nuts, seeds, and grains. It is an important component of the diet and helps to maintain bone health. It is also necessary for the production of proteins, fats, and carbohydrates. In terms of nutrition, phosphorus is found in large amounts in meat, poultry, fish, and dairy products, and in smaller amounts in plant-based foods. The daily recommended intake of phosphorus is 700 mg for adults. Phosphorus is an essential element that is essential for human health. It is important for the development and maintenance of healthy bones and teeth, as well as for many metabolic processes.

Phosphorus is an essential mineral nutrient found in the body, which plays a vital role in many bodily processes. It is a major component of bones and teeth, and helps to regulate metabolism, energy production, and cell growth and repair. Phosphorus also plays a role in nerve impulse transmission, muscle contraction, and kidney function. In addition to its role in the body's structure, phosphorus is required for the formation of DNA and RNA, which are essential for cell growth and repair. It also helps to regulate the acid-base balance in the body and is involved in many biochemical reactions. In terms of its nutritional benefits, phosphorus helps to maintain strong bones and teeth, and is also important for the absorption and use of other minerals, such as calcium and magnesium. It also helps to maintain healthy blood pressure and cholesterol levels and may reduce the risk of developing certain types of cancer. Phosphorus is found in many foods, such as dairy products, eggs, fish, meat, poultry, and certain grains and legumes. It is also found in certain vitamins and supplements, such as multivitamins. For those who may be deficient in phosphorus, supplementation may be necessary. Overall, phosphorus is an important mineral for the body, helping to regulate metabolism, energy production, and cell growth and repair. It also helps to maintain strong bones and teeth and may reduce the risk of certain types of cancer. For those who may be deficient in phosphorus, supplementation may be necessary.

Food sources

Phosphorus is an essential mineral for the human body. It plays an important role in many biological processes, such as energy production, cell growth, and maintenance of bones and teeth. Because of this, it's important to get enough phosphorus in your diet. There are many foods that are excellent sources of phosphorus.

Meat: Phosphorus is an important element found in meat, and it plays a critical role in the human body. It is a mineral that is essential for healthy bones and teeth, as well as for the production of energy from carbohydrates and fats. Phosphorus is also important for muscle contraction and nerve function, as well as for the release of hormones such as insulin. Phosphorus is naturally present in many foods, including meat. It is found in larger amounts in red meats such as beef, lamb, and pork, as well as in chicken and turkey. It is also found in smaller amounts in fish and eggs. Processed meats such as sausages, hot dogs, and bacon also contain phosphorus, although in much lower amounts. The recommended daily intake of phosphorus for adults is 700 mg and should come from a variety of foods. Eating a balanced diet that includes meat can help to ensure that your phosphorus requirements are met. It is important to note that excessive phosphorus intake can lead to health problems, so it is important to follow the recommended intake. In addition to its role in the body, phosphorus is also important for the production of proteins and is a key component in the production of DNA. Phosphorus also plays an important role in the absorption of other minerals, such as calcium and magnesium, which are both essential for healthy bones and teeth. When it comes to nutrition, phosphorus is an important part of a healthy diet. Eating a balanced diet that includes meat can help to ensure that your phosphorus requirements are met. It is important to note that excessive phosphorus intake can lead to health problems, so it is important to follow the recommended intake.

Poultry: Poultry is a great source of phosphorus. It is found in the bones, skin, and other tissues of birds. The amount of phosphorus in poultry can vary depending on the part of the bird. For example, the breast meat contains the highest amount of phosphorus, whereas the leg meat has the lowest amount. When it comes to nutrition for poultry, phosphorus plays an important role. It helps to provide energy for growth and development and is also essential for maintaining strong bones and teeth. In addition, phosphorus helps to maintain a healthy digestive system and regulates the body's acid-base balance. The recommended daily intake of phosphorus for poultry is 0.3 to 0.5 grams per kg of body weight. This amount should be divided into two or three meals. It's important to make sure the poultry is getting enough phosphorus, as too little can lead to poor growth and development. When feeding poultry, it's important to provide a balanced diet that contains adequate amounts of phosphorus. This can be done by feeding a commercially prepared feed that contains a proper balance of vitamins and minerals, including phosphorus. Additionally, poultry can benefit from occasional treats, such as fresh fruits and vegetables, which also contain phosphorus. In conclusion, phosphorus is an essential mineral found in poultry that helps to provide nutritional support for a variety of physiological processes. It is found in the bones, skin, and other tissues of birds, and is necessary for normal growth and development. The recommended daily intake of phosphorus for poultry is 0.3 to 0.5 grams per kg of body weight and should be divided into two or three meals. By providing a balanced diet that contains adequate amounts of phosphorus, poultry can benefit from the nutritional support it provides.

Eggs: Phosphorus is an important mineral found in eggs that plays an important role in many bodily functions. It is an essential component of DNA, RNA and phospholipids, which are important components of cell membranes. It is also found in important enzymes and hormones. Phosphorus helps to form bones and teeth and is important for the absorption of calcium and other minerals. Additionally, it is an important component in cell energy production. Eggs provide a good source of phosphorus, with one large egg containing about 85 milligrams. This amount is about 10 percent of the recommended daily intake for adults. Additionally, eggs are a good source of protein, which helps to maintain healthy muscles. Eggs are an easy and convenient way to get phosphorus, as well as other important nutrients. They can be cooked in a variety of ways, such as boiled, scrambled, poached or baked. Additionally, they can be added to salads or sandwiches, or used as an ingredient in baking. Eating a healthy and balanced diet that includes a variety of foods is the best way to get all the essential nutrients, including phosphorus. However, if you are not getting enough phosphorus from your diet, you may want to consider taking a supplement. Additionally, it is important to talk to your doctor before taking any supplements, as too much phosphorus can lead to health problems. Overall, eggs are a great source of phosphorus, as well as other important nutrients. They are an easy and convenient way to get the phosphorus your body needs, as well as other important vitamins and minerals. Eating a healthy and balanced diet that includes a variety of foods is the best way to ensure you are getting all the essential nutrients your body needs.

Fish: Phosphorus is an essential element for all living things and is found in fish in the form of phosphate. It plays a key role in the development and maintenance of a healthy fish population. Phosphorus is found in the muscles, bones, fins, and scales of fish, and it is essential for their growth and development. Phosphorus helps to regulate the acid-base balance in fish, as well as playing a role in the metabolism of proteins, carbohydrates, and lipids. Phosphorus is a major component of the diet of fish, and it is found in the aquatic food chain. Phytoplankton, the base of the aquatic food chain, contain high levels of phosphorus, and this phosphorus is then passed through the food chain, eventually ending up in the bodies of fish. However, the levels of phosphorus found in fish can vary greatly depending on the species, their diet, and their environment. The amount of phosphorus in a fish's diet is important for their health, as it helps to ensure that the fish's body has all the nutrients it needs to grow and develop properly. If a fish does not have enough phosphorus in its diet, it can lead to stunted growth and poor health. On the other hand, if a fish has too much phosphorus in its diet, it can lead to problems such as increased levels of phosphorus in the water, which can lead to eutrophication. Therefore, it is important for fish to have the right balance of phosphorus in their diet. Too much phosphorus can lead to eutrophication, while not enough can lead to stunted growth. Fish farmers should carefully monitor the levels of phosphorus in the diets of their fish and make any necessary adjustments to ensure that the fish have the right balance of nutrients. In summary, phosphorus is an essential element for all living things, and it is found in fish in the form of phosphate. Phosphorus plays a key role in the growth and development of fish, and it is found in the aquatic food chain. It is important for fish to have the right balance of phosphorus in their diet, as too much can lead to eutrophication, while too little can lead to stunted growth. Fish farmers should carefully monitor the levels of phosphorus in the diets of their fish and make any necessary adjustments to ensure that the fish have the right balance of nutrients.

Grains: Phosphorus is an essential element for the growth and development of most crops, including grains. It is found in the soil and is taken up by plants as they grow, but it can also be added to the soil in the form of fertilizer. When phosphorus is applied to the soil, it helps to increase crop yields and improve the overall quality of the grain, as well as helping to reduce disease and insect infestations. Phosphorus is a major component of the cell walls of the grains, and it helps to strengthen the cell walls and keep them from breaking down. It also helps to increase the availability of other essential nutrients, such as nitrogen, potassium, and calcium, which are important for the growth and development of the grain. Phosphorus also helps to improve the water-holding capacity of the soil, which can help to improve the overall health of the soil and the crop. Phosphorus is also important for the production of carbohydrates and proteins. When it is added to the soil, it helps to increase the amount of carbohydrates and proteins in the grain, which helps to improve the nutritional value of the grain. Additionally, phosphorus can help to reduce the amount of toxins in the grain, which can help to reduce the risk of food-borne illnesses. In addition to its role in crop production, phosphorus is also important for the environment. It helps to reduce soil erosion, improve soil fertility, and reduce the amount of pollutants in the environment. It also helps to improve the quality of water, air, and soil. Overall, phosphorus is an essential element for the growth and development of grains. It helps to strengthen the cell walls of the grains, increase their nutritional value, and reduce the amount of pollutants in the environment. Without phosphorus, grains would not be able to grow and produce the high-quality grain that we need to feed ourselves and the world.

Legumes: Phosphorus is an essential macronutrient that plays a major role in plant growth and development. Legumes, such as peas, beans, lentils, and chickpeas, are rich sources of phosphorus and many other essential minerals and vitamins. Phosphorus is a macronutrient necessary for plant growth, development, and metabolic processes. It is involved in energy transfer, photosynthesis, and cell membrane formation and helps with the absorption and utilization of other vital nutrients. Legumes are packed with phosphorus, providing a valuable source of this nutrient for human and animal diets. A half-cup serving of cooked beans, peas, lentils, or chickpeas can provide up to 20% of the recommended daily intake of phosphorus. Phosphorus is important for the development and maintenance of strong, healthy bones and teeth. It also helps to regulate kidney and heart functions and aids in muscle contractions. Phosphorus is also essential for the production of ATP, an energy molecule used by cells to carry out all metabolic processes. Legumes are also a great source of other essential minerals and vitamins, such as iron, potassium, magnesium, zinc, and B-vitamins. These nutrients help to support overall health and wellness and can help to reduce the risk of certain chronic diseases. In addition to their high nutrient content, legumes are low in fat, rich in dietary fibre, and high in protein. They are also incredibly versatile and can be used in a variety of dishes, from soups and stews to salads and side dishes. All in all, legumes are an excellent source of phosphorus and other essential vitamins and minerals. Including them in your diet can help to ensure that you are getting the nutrients you need to support good health.

Magnesium

Magnesium is an essential mineral found in many foods and is a vital component in many metabolic processes. It plays a role in more than 300 enzymatic reactions, including those involved with energy production, protein synthesis, and DNA and RNA synthesis. Magnesium is also important for bone health, muscle contraction, nerve transmission, and blood sugar control. Foods that are high in magnesium include legumes, nuts, seeds, whole grains, dark leafy greens, and dairy products. Magnesium is also found in certain fruits, vegetables, and even some fortified foods, such as breakfast cereals and some types of breads. Legumes are one of the best sources of magnesium. They are packed with magnesium, as well as other essential minerals, vitamins, and fibre. Among the legumes that are highest in magnesium are black beans, kidney beans, navy beans, lima beans, and lentils. Nuts and seeds are also good sources of magnesium. Almonds, Brazil nuts, cashews, pine nuts, and pumpkin seeds are among the best sources. They also contain other essential vitamins, minerals, and healthy fats. Whole grains are also a good source of magnesium. Whole grain bread, brown rice, quinoa, oats, and buckwheat are all good choices. These grains are also high in other essential nutrients, such as fibre, iron, B vitamins, and zinc. Dark, leafy greens are also rich in magnesium. Spinach, kale, Swiss chard, and collard greens are some of the best sources. They are also high in other important minerals and vitamins, such as calcium, iron, and vitamin K. Dairy products are also good sources of magnesium, although they are not as high in magnesium as other foods. Milk, yogurt, and cheese are all good sources. Fortified foods are also an excellent source of magnesium. Some breakfast cereals and breads are fortified with magnesium, as well as other essential vitamins and minerals. Magnesium is an important mineral that plays a role in many metabolic processes, including energy production, protein synthesis, and nerve transmission. Eating a variety of foods that are high in magnesium, such as legumes, nuts, seeds, whole grains, dark leafy greens, dairy, and fortified foods, is the best way to ensure adequate intake.

Magnesium is a mineral that is vital for the body's health and well-being. It is involved in over 300 biochemical processes in the body, including the formation of bones and teeth, muscle and nerve function, energy production and metabolism, and the maintenance of proper blood pressure and blood sugar levels. Magnesium helps to relax the muscles and nerves and is a key component in the body's energy production. Its involvement in energy production makes it essential for athletes and those who engage in regular physical activity. It is also important for mental health and can help reduce anxiety and stress. Magnesium is also important for the heart. It helps to regulate the heart's rhythm and maintain normal blood pressure. It also helps to reduce the risk of stroke, heart attack, and other cardiovascular diseases. Magnesium is involved in the formation of bones and teeth and is necessary for healthy bone density. It is important for the formation of collagen, which helps to keep skin healthy and looking young. It is also involved in the metabolism of carbohydrates, fats, and proteins, which are all important for overall health. In addition, magnesium helps to maintain healthy levels of certain hormones in the body, such as insulin, which helps to regulate blood sugar levels. It also helps to reduce inflammation, which can be beneficial for those suffering from arthritis, asthma, and other inflammatory conditions. Finally, magnesium is important for the absorption of other essential vitamins and minerals, such as calcium and potassium. A magnesium deficiency can lead to a variety of health problems, so it is important to make sure you get enough of this important nutrient in your diet. Overall, magnesium is a key mineral for the body's health and well-being. It is involved in a variety of biochemical processes, helps to maintain healthy bones, teeth, and skin, and is important for energy production, mental health, and the absorption of other essential vitamins and minerals.

Food sources

Magnesium is an essential mineral found in many foods and is important for many bodily functions.

Pumpkin Seeds: Pumpkin seeds are a powerhouse of nutrition, packed with essential vitamins, minerals, and compounds that can benefit the health of your body. One of the most prominent minerals in pumpkin seeds is magnesium. Magnesium is a mineral that is essential for the proper functioning of the human body. It is involved in hundreds of processes, including the metabolism of fat, carbohydrates, and proteins, as well as the production of energy and the formation of bone and muscle tissue. It also helps to regulate blood pressure, prevent muscle cramps, and maintain nerve and muscle function. Magnesium is found in many foods, including green vegetables, nuts, and seeds. Pumpkin seeds are a particularly good source of magnesium, providing about 37 mg per 1-ounce serving. This is almost 10% of the recommended daily allowance (RDA) for magnesium. The magnesium in pumpkin seeds can help to reduce stress and anxiety, improve sleep quality, and boost energy levels. It is also thought to help reduce the risk of type-2 diabetes, high blood pressure, and cardiovascular disease. In addition, research suggests that magnesium may be beneficial for those with migraines, premenstrual syndrome, and depression. Pumpkin seeds are also high in healthy fats, which can help to reduce inflammation and reduce the risk of certain diseases. They are also a good source of plant-based protein, as well as vitamins A, C, and E, and a variety of antioxidants. To reap the benefits of the magnesium in pumpkin seeds, it is best to consume them in their raw, unsalted form. They can be eaten as a snack, added to salads, or sprinkled on oatmeal or yogurt. They can also be roasted and used as a crunchy topping for soups and stews. In conclusion, pumpkin seeds are an excellent source of magnesium, a mineral that is essential for many body processes. Eating pumpkin seeds as part of a healthy diet can help to reduce stress and anxiety, improve sleep quality, and boost energy levels. They are also a good source of healthy fats, plant-based protein, vitamins, and antioxidants.

Chia Seeds: Chia seeds are considered a superfood due to their high nutrient content. One of the key components of chia seeds is magnesium, an essential mineral for overall health and wellness. Magnesium is involved in more than 300 enzymatic reactions in the body, making it essential for energy production, protein synthesis, blood sugar regulation, and muscle and nerve function. It is also important for strong bones and teeth, healthy skin, and normal heart rhythms. Chia seeds are an excellent source of dietary magnesium. One ounce of chia seeds contains approximately 49 milligrams of magnesium, which is about 10-12% of the recommended daily intake. This makes chia seeds a great option for those looking to increase their dietary magnesium intake. In addition to magnesium, chia seeds are also a good source of other minerals like calcium, phosphorus, and zinc. They are also rich in antioxidants, omega-3 fatty acids, dietary fibre, and protein. Studies have shown that consuming chia seeds may help reduce inflammation, improve heart health, and lower blood pressure. They may also help boost energy levels and improve exercise performance by providing a slow and steady release of energy. Overall, chia seeds are an excellent source of magnesium and other essential nutrients. They are easy to incorporate into your diet and can be eaten either raw, soaked, or ground into some flour. Adding chia seeds to your diet may help promote overall health and wellness.

Almonds: Almonds are one of the most nutritious and versatile nuts, and they are high in magnesium. Almonds are a great source of magnesium, providing 19% of the daily value in just one serving. The main function of magnesium is to help the body absorb calcium, which is essential for healthy bones and teeth. It also helps to regulate nerve and muscle function, as well as the heart rhythm. Magnesium is involved in energy production, and its presence helps to convert food into energy. It also helps to regulate blood sugar levels, reducing the risk of diabetes. Almonds are a great source of magnesium, and it is easy to incorporate them into your diet. They can be eaten as a snack, added to salads, or used in baking. Almonds are also full of healthy fats, protein, and dietary fibre, making them a nutritious and filling snack. Magnesium is an essential mineral that is involved in many bodily processes. Almonds are a great source of magnesium, providing 19% of the daily value in just one serving. Eating almonds regularly can help to ensure that your body is getting enough magnesium, which can help to regulate nerve and muscle function, maintain strong bones, control blood sugar levels, and help to convert food into energy.

Spinach: Spinach is a popular green leafy vegetable that is full of essential nutrients. One of the most important nutrients in spinach is magnesium. One cup of cooked spinach contains 157 milligrams of magnesium, which is almost 40% of the recommended daily allowance for adults. Magnesium is also found in other dark green vegetables, legumes, nuts, and whole grains. Magnesium is important for many body functions, but it also has some important health benefits. For example, it can help to reduce inflammation, which is associated with many chronic diseases such as heart disease, diabetes, and arthritis. It can also reduce the risk of stroke and help to protect against some types of cancer. Magnesium is also important for mental health. It can reduce the symptoms of depression and anxiety and can help to improve cognitive function. It can also help to reduce the risk of Alzheimer's disease and dementia. In addition to its health benefits, magnesium is also important for athletes. It helps to maintain muscle and nerve function, which can improve performance and reduce fatigue. It can also help to improve post-workout recovery. Overall, magnesium is an essential nutrient that is found in many foods, but spinach is especially high in it. Eating spinach can help to provide your body with the magnesium it needs for many important functions and can also help to reduce the risk of certain chronic diseases and improve mental health. So, make sure to include spinach in your diet for the many benefits it provides.

Cashews: Cashews are a popular snack food and a great source of magnesium. One ounce of cashews contains 83 milligrams of magnesium. This is about 22 percent of the recommended daily value. This amount of magnesium is enough to provide the body with the necessary amount of the mineral to support its vital processes. Cashews are also a great source of other minerals, including potassium, phosphorus, and zinc. These minerals help to regulate blood pressure, support the development of strong bones, and protect the body from disease. In addition, cashews are high in healthy monounsaturated and polyunsaturated fats. These fats help to lower bad cholesterol levels and reduce the risk of heart disease. Magnesium is also important for mental health. It helps to reduce stress, anxiety, and depression. Magnesium also supports healthy sleep cycles, which are essential for overall wellbeing. Eating cashews can help to provide the body with the necessary magnesium to support these mental health benefits. Cashews are a great way to get the necessary magnesium for the body's vital processes. They are also a great source of other minerals, healthy fats, and mental health benefits. Eating cashews is an easy and tasty way to ensure that the body is getting enough of this essential mineral.

Peanuts: Peanuts are a popular snack food, and for good reason. Not only are they tasty and convenient, but they are also packed with beneficial nutrients. One of those nutrients is magnesium, an essential mineral that is important for a number of bodily functions. A one ounce serving of peanuts contains about 25 milligrams of magnesium, or about seven percent of the daily recommended value for adults. This is a significant amount of magnesium, considering that most other nuts only contain about two to four percent of the daily value. In addition to magnesium, peanuts are also rich in other important nutrients, including protein, fibre, and healthy fats. They are also a good source of antioxidants, which can help protect the body from free radical damage. The health benefits associated with peanuts are numerous. Overall, peanuts are a nutritious snack that can be enjoyed in moderation. The magnesium present in peanuts can provide a number of health benefits, making them an even better choice. So if you're looking for a nutritious snack, look no further than peanuts.

Soy milk: Soy milk is a popular plant-based milk alternative that is made from soybeans. It has become a popular choice for those looking to reduce their dairy consumption or avoid animal-based products. While soy milk is a great source of vitamins and minerals, it is also an important source of magnesium. Soy milk is a particularly good source of magnesium, with one cup providing around 24% of the daily recommended intake. Soy milk is also fortified with other essential vitamins and minerals, including calcium, vitamin D, and vitamin B12. It is low in fat and calories and is a great choice for those looking to reduce their cholesterol or manage their weight. Soy milk is an excellent alternative to dairy milk and is a great source of magnesium. It is low in fat and calories and is fortified with other essential vitamins and minerals. It is a great choice for those looking to reduce their dairy consumption or manage their weight. For those looking to get their daily recommended intake of magnesium, soy milk is an excellent option.

Oats: Oats are a great source of magnesium, with one cup providing around 39% of the recommended daily amount. It's also found in a range of other grains and cereals, as well as nuts, legumes, and some vegetables. The role of magnesium in the body is extensive. It's involved in energy production, muscle and nerve function, and helps to regulate blood pressure. It's also essential for the formation of bones and teeth and helps to keep the heart rhythm regular. Magnesium also plays a role in immune function and helps to reduce inflammation. Getting enough magnesium is important for overall health, however deficiency can lead to a range of issues. These can include fatigue, muscle cramps, poor concentration, and poor sleep quality. It's estimated that around two thirds of the population don't get enough magnesium in their diet. Including oats in your diet is an easy way to increase your magnesium intake. Oats are also rich in other essential nutrients, such as protein, fibre, B vitamins, and iron. They're versatile and can be included in a range of meals and snacks. Making oatmeal is an easy way to get your daily dose of magnesium. It's also a great option for breakfast, as it's filling and can help to keep you energized throughout the day. Adding nuts, seeds, and fresh fruit to your oatmeal is a great way to boost the nutritional content even further. Including oats in your diet is a great way to make sure you're getting enough magnesium. It's an essential mineral that plays an important role in many processes in the body. Getting enough magnesium can help to keep you feeling energized and healthy.

Chloride

Chloride is an essential mineral found in many foods. It is a major component of table salt, and it is also found naturally in many foods, including dairy products, meats, fish, poultry, eggs, some fruits and vegetables, and grains. Chloride helps keep the body's acid-base balance, aids in digestion, and helps transport other minerals and nutrients throughout the body. Chloride is an essential mineral that helps keep the body's acid-base balance. The body needs a certain amount of chloride to help keep its pH levels balanced, which is important for many bodily functions. Chloride also helps with digestion by aiding in the breakdown of food, and it helps transport other minerals and nutrients throughout the body. Chloride is generally found in three forms in food: chloride salts, chloride ions, and chloride compounds. Chloride salts are the most common form found in food and are usually found in the form of table salt. Chloride ions are found in certain fruits and vegetables, such as oranges, lemons, and potatoes, while chloride compounds are found in dairy products, meats, fish, poultry, and eggs. The body needs a certain amount of chloride to stay healthy, but it is important to not consume too much as too much chloride can lead to an imbalance in the body's acid-base balance, which can be dangerous. The recommended daily intake of chloride for adults is 2.3-3.6 grams per day, depending on age and gender. Chloride can also be found in some processed foods, such as canned foods and processed meats, but these foods should be consumed in moderation due to the high levels of salt and other additives. In conclusion, chloride is an essential mineral that helps keep the body's acid-base balance, aids in digestion, and helps transport other minerals and nutrients throughout the body. It is found naturally in many foods, including dairy products, meats, fish, poultry, eggs, some fruits and vegetables, and grains. It is important to not consume too much chloride, as too much can lead to an imbalance in the body's acid-base balance.

Chloride is a necessary part of everyday health and well-being. It is an essential electrolyte that helps regulate the balance of fluids in the body, playing an important role in the maintenance of healthy blood pressure and other bodily functions. Chloride is found in the body in the form of chloride ions, which are important for the regulation of sodium and potassium levels in the body, allowing for the proper function of nerves, muscles, digestion and other important bodily processes. Chloride is also important for the formation of hydrochloric acid in the stomach, which is essential for the digestion of food. Chloride is also essential for the body's ability to absorb vitamins and minerals. It helps the body break down and absorb nutrients from food and helps the body regulate the amount of water in the body. Chloride also helps the body maintain a neutral pH balance, which is essential for proper functioning of bodily systems. Chloride is also important for the body's natural defence system. It helps the body fight off bacteria and other harmful organisms by acting as an antiseptic. It also helps the body to rid itself of toxins and waste products, preventing the build-up of harmful substances in the body. Chloride is also important for maintaining healthy bones and teeth. It helps the body to absorb calcium, which is essential for bone health. It also helps to keep the teeth and gums healthy by preventing tooth decay and other dental problems. Overall, chloride is essential for the body's overall health and well-being. It helps the body to function properly, absorb nutrients, defend against bacteria, and maintain healthy bones and teeth. Without sufficient chloride in the body, a person may suffer from a variety of health problems. For this reason, it is important to ensure that you are getting enough chloride in your diet.

Food sources

Chloride is an essential electrolyte for the human body found naturally in a variety of foods.

Seaweed: Chloride is an essential mineral for the health of humans and animals, and it also plays an important role in the growth of aquatic plants, such as seaweed. Seaweed is a type of marine algae that is rich in a variety of minerals and vitamins, including chloride. Chloride is essential for the proper functioning of cells, including those of the nervous system, and is also a key component of stomach acid, which helps to break down food. Chloride is found in seawater, and it is taken up by seaweed during photosynthesis. Seaweed is a major source of dietary chloride for humans and animals, and it is particularly important for those who live near the ocean and consume seaweed as part of their regular diet. Seaweed is rich in a variety of minerals and vitamins, including chloride, which helps to support overall health and well-being. Chloride plays an important role in the growth of seaweed, as it helps to maintain the proper balance of ions in the water surrounding the seaweed. Without adequate chloride, the seaweed may not be able to obtain the necessary nutrients for growth and development. Additionally, chloride helps to regulate the pH of the water, which is important for the growth of seaweed. Chloride also helps to protect seaweed from environmental stressors, such as high temperatures and ultraviolet radiation. When seaweed is exposed to these stresses, chloride helps to stabilize the cells of the seaweed and protect them from damage. In addition to its role in growth and protection of seaweed, chloride also helps to promote the growth of beneficial bacteria, which help to keep the seaweed healthy. These bacteria play an important role in the breakdown of organic matter and the removal of pollutants from the water. In conclusion, chloride is an important mineral for the health of humans and animals, and it is also essential for the growth and protection of seaweed. Seaweed is a major source of dietary chloride, and its consumption is important for those who live near the ocean and consume seaweed as part of their regular diet. Seaweed is rich in a variety of minerals and vitamins, including chloride, which helps to support overall health and well-being.

Tomatoes: Tomatoes are a popular fruit found in many kitchens around the world. They are a beneficial source of vitamins, minerals, and antioxidants and are a key ingredient in many dishes. One mineral found in tomatoes is chloride, an electrolyte important for maintaining fluid balance and maintaining the proper functioning of the nervous system. Chloride is a component of the molecule chloride ion, which is an electrolyte found in the body and is important for regulating the amount of water in the body. It also helps to maintain the proper pH balance in the body and helps to transport nutrients and waste products. Chloride is found in a variety of foods, including tomatoes. Tomatoes contain a moderate amount of chloride, with a one-cup serving providing about 11 milligrams of chloride. This amount is roughly equivalent to the amount of chloride found in other foods like potatoes and bananas. Chloride plays an important role in maintaining the proper functioning of the nervous system, as it helps to conduct electrical signals throughout the body. It is also important for maintaining fluid balance, as it helps to regulate the amount of water in the body. Chloride also helps to transport nutrients and waste products throughout the body. Eating a diet rich in chloride can help to maintain the proper functioning of the nervous system and fluid balance and can help to transport nutrients and waste products throughout the body. Tomatoes are an excellent source of chloride and can be eaten as part of a healthy diet.

Lettuce: Lettuce is a good source of chloride, containing approximately 25 to 30 milligrams per one-cup serving. This amount of chloride provides approximately 1.3 to 1.5 percent of the recommended daily intake of chloride for adults. While this may not seem like a lot, it can still contribute significantly to the body's overall chloride needs. Chloride is necessary for the body to properly digest food and absorb nutrients. It is also important for maintaining the proper balance of electrolytes in the body, which helps to regulate heart rate and blood pressure. Additionally, chloride helps to regulate nerve impulses, muscle contractions, and blood pH. Chloride is also necessary for the body to produce hydrochloric acid, which is important for breaking down food in the stomach. This acid also helps to absorb vitamins and minerals from food, as well as protect against harmful bacteria and other pathogens. The primary benefit of consuming chloride through lettuce is its ability to help maintain the body's balance of electrolytes. This can help to lower blood pressure and improve heart health. Additionally, it can help to prevent dehydration, as well as improve digestion and nutrient absorption. Overall, lettuce is a healthy, nutrient-dense food that is an excellent source of chloride. Eating lettuce can help to maintain the body's internal balance, improve heart health, and aid in digestion and nutrient absorption. Therefore, consuming lettuce is a great way to ensure that the body is receiving an adequate amount of chloride.

Celery: Chloride is an important mineral found in celery that plays an important role in the body. Celery is a great source of chloride, providing about 40mg per cup. This can be beneficial for those who are deficient in chloride, which can lead to a variety of health problems. Chloride deficiencies can cause fatigue, muscle weakness, and increased risk of infection, and can lead to electrolyte imbalances. Celery is an excellent source of chloride and can be beneficial for those who are deficient in this important mineral.

Olives: Chloride is an essential mineral that is found in olives, with olives having some of the highest chloride levels among other fruits and vegetables. It is found in the brine solution that is used to preserve olives, as well as in the olive itself. The amount of chloride in olives can vary depending on how they are processed and stored. Generally, olives that are stored in brine have higher levels of chloride than those that are canned or jarred, as the brine helps to preserve the olives. Olives are also a good source of dietary fibre, which can help to reduce cholesterol levels and improve digestion. Fibre also helps to keep the digestive system healthy. Overall, chloride is an essential mineral that is found in olives and is important for the proper functioning of the body. It is also a good source of dietary fibre, which can help to reduce cholesterol levels and improve digestion.

Sodium

Sodium is an essential nutrient found in many foods. It helps the body maintain the correct balance of fluids and electrolytes, aids in nerve transmission and muscle contraction, and is required for normal heart and kidney functioning. It is also necessary for proper digestion and absorption of food. However, too much sodium can be unhealthy. The average American consumes more than 3,400 milligrams of sodium every day—almost double the recommended daily allowance of 2,300 milligrams. Too much sodium can lead to high blood pressure, an increased risk of stroke, and other health problems. Fortunately, there are plenty of ways to get the right amount of sodium in your diet without overdoing it. Eating a diet rich in fresh fruits and vegetables, whole grains, and lean proteins is a great place to start. These foods are naturally low in sodium and provide many essential vitamins and minerals. In addition, there are a variety of low-sodium options available for those looking to reduce their sodium intake. Low-sodium soups, vegetables, and canned foods are widely available and can help lower your daily sodium intake. For those looking to add flavour to their meals without overdoing the sodium, there are a number of alternatives. Herbs, spices, and citrus juices are all great options that can add flavour without adding a lot of sodium. Finally, many processed foods are high in sodium. For example, canned soups, frozen dinners, and packaged snacks are often loaded with sodium. Reading nutrition labels can help you identify high-sodium products and opt for healthier alternatives. By making smart food choices and limiting processed foods, you can ensure you're getting the right amount of sodium in your diet. Eating a diet rich in fresh, whole foods and limiting your processed food intake can help you avoid too much sodium and keep your health on track.

Sodium is an essential mineral that our bodies need in order to function properly. It is a vital component of bodily fluids, including blood and plasma, and it helps regulate blood pressure and maintain healthy nerve and muscle function. Sodium also helps to balance the acid-base balance in our bodies and is essential for proper hydration. Sodium plays a key role in nerve impulse transmission and muscle contraction. It helps to regulate the amount of water in and around cells, which is important for maintaining normal physical and mental health. Sodium also helps to move nutrients into cells and waste products out of cells, which is important for digestion and absorption of food. Sodium is also important for maintaining healthy blood pressure. It helps to regulate the balance of salt and water in the body, which helps to keep blood pressure in a normal range. Too much sodium can lead to high blood pressure, which can increase the risk of stroke, heart attack, and other cardiovascular problems. Too little sodium can lead to low blood pressure, which can cause fatigue, dizziness, and fainting. Finally, sodium helps to regulate body temperature, which is important for maintaining a normal body temperature. In addition, sodium helps to keep bones strong by helping to regulate the balance of calcium and phosphate in the body. Overall, sodium is an essential mineral that plays a key role in maintaining normal bodily functions. It is important to ensure that you are getting enough sodium in your diet to prevent health problems. Too much or too little sodium can lead to serious health problems, so it is important to consume it in moderation.

Keeping the balance

Maintaining a balanced sodium level in the body is critical for overall health. Sodium is an essential electrolyte that helps regulate the balance of fluids in the body and is necessary for proper functioning of nerves and muscles. It is also important for maintaining blood pressure and healthy hydration levels. When the body's sodium levels become too high or too low, it can cause a variety of health problems. High sodium levels in the body can lead to an increased risk of stroke, heart disease, and hypertension. An excess of sodium can also cause fluid retention, which can lead to swelling in the hands, feet, and ankles. Too much sodium can also upset the body's acid-base balance and result in headaches, nausea, and fatigue. On the other hand, having too little sodium in the body can cause hyponatremia, a condition in which the sodium levels in the blood are too low. This can lead to confusion, muscle weakness, seizures, coma, and even death. In order to maintain a healthy sodium balance, it is important to follow a balanced diet and to eat a variety of foods that are low in sodium. This includes avoiding processed foods and fast food, as well as reducing the amount of salt added to food during cooking and at the table. It is also important to stay hydrated by drinking plenty of water throughout the day. Keeping the sodium level balanced is essential for maintaining overall health. By eating a balanced diet and limiting processed foods and added salt, individuals can help ensure their sodium levels remain within the normal range and avoid the health risks associated with high or low sodium levels.

The difference between sea salt and table salt

Salt is a mineral composed primarily of sodium chloride (NaCl). It is found in abundance in both the ocean and in underground deposits. The major difference between sea and table salt is the amount of processing each undergoes. Sea salt is harvested from evaporated ocean water or from underground salt deposits. It is often left unrefined and may contain trace amounts of minerals and other elements. Sea salt is usually coarser than table salt and has a stronger flavour. Table salt is mined from underground salt deposits or evaporated sea water. It is then heavily processed, removing any minerals or other elements. It is then iodized, meaning iodine is added to it, which helps to prevent iodine deficiency disorders. Table salt is much finer than sea salt and has a less intense flavour. In terms of sodium, sea salt and table salt have similar amounts of sodium by weight. However, due to the difference in grain size, the amount of sodium in a teaspoon of sea salt is actually less than a teaspoon of table salt. A teaspoon of table salt contains about 40% more sodium than a teaspoon of sea salt. In conclusion, sea and table salt are both composed primarily of sodium chloride, but the difference in processing creates a difference in flavour, texture, and sodium content. Sea salt is coarser and has a more intense flavour, while table salt is more refined and has a milder flavour. In terms of sodium, a teaspoon of table salt contains more sodium than a teaspoon of sea salt.

Natural food sources

Eggs: Sodium is an important mineral that is found in many different foods, including eggs. Eggs are a great source of protein and other nutrients, but they also contain significant amounts of sodium. While eggs are not considered to be unhealthy, they are high in sodium, and it is important to be aware of this when planning meals. The average egg contains around 70mg of sodium, or 3% of the daily recommended value. This may not seem like a lot, but it can quickly add up. For example, if you have three eggs for breakfast, you are already consuming 210mg of sodium. Sodium is an essential nutrient for the body, but too much of it can be harmful to health. Too much sodium can increase blood pressure, which can lead to heart disease and stroke. It is important to keep sodium intake within the recommended limits of 2,300mg per day. Eggs can be a great source of nutritious protein, but they should be consumed in moderation. Eating just one or two eggs per day can provide a healthy amount of protein and other nutrients, while still keeping sodium intake within the recommended limits. In addition to eating fewer eggs, there are other ways to reduce sodium in the diet. Eating more fresh fruits and vegetables, choosing lean proteins, and avoiding processed foods can all help to reduce sodium intake. In conclusion, while eggs are a great source of protein and other important nutrients, they can also be high in sodium. Eating them in moderation and making other dietary changes can help to keep sodium intake within the recommended limits.

Legumes: Legumes are a type of plant-based food that are commonly used in many different cultures around the world. They are a great source of protein, fibre, and other essential nutrients. Legumes are also low in calories and fat, making them a healthy option for those looking to lose weight. However, legumes can also be high in sodium, which can be a concern for those who have high blood pressure or are at risk for heart disease. A healthy diet typically consists of no more than 2,300 milligrams of sodium per day, with some people needing to limit their intake even further. Legumes can range from low too high in sodium content, depending on the variety. Common types of legumes that are lower in sodium include black beans, kidney beans, and chickpeas. These types of legumes contain about 10 to 15 milligrams of sodium per serving. On the other hand, canned legumes can be significantly higher in sodium. For example, canned black beans contain about 180 milligrams of sodium per serving, while canned chickpeas contain about 250 milligrams per serving. When preparing legumes at home, it is important to pay attention to the sodium content. If a recipe calls for canned beans or other canned legumes, drain and rinse them before using to reduce the sodium content. Additionally, adding spices and herbs can help to reduce the need for added salt. In conclusion, legumes can be a healthy and nutritious addition to any diet. While most types of legumes are relatively low in sodium, it is important to keep an eye on the sodium content of canned legumes and to use low-sodium alternatives whenever possible.

Nuts: Nuts are a great source of nutrition and are an important part of a healthy diet. They are high in healthy fats, protein, and a variety of vitamins and minerals. One of the minerals found in nuts is sodium. Most types of nuts contain small amounts of sodium, generally ranging from 0-15 milligrams (mg) per one ounce serving. Almonds are one of the lowest-sodium nuts, with just 1 mg per ounce. Cashews, pecans, walnuts, and macadamia nuts all contain around 4-5 mg per ounce. Pistachios and sunflower seeds contain a bit more, with around 8-10 mg per ounce. The sodium content of nuts can be increased if they are roasted in salt or if they are purchased in a salted variety. This is why it is important to read nutrition labels when purchasing nuts to ensure you are not consuming too much sodium. Nuts are a great way to get some extra nutrition into your diet, and their sodium content is relatively low. However, it is still important to monitor the amount of sodium you are consuming from all sources, including nuts, to ensure that you are not exceeding the recommended daily limit. Eating a variety of nuts, in moderation, is the best way to ensure you are getting the benefits of the nutrients without consuming too much sodium.

Salmon: Salmon is a healthy, nutrient-rich fish that is a popular choice for many diets. Not only is it a great source of lean protein, but it is also packed with vitamins, minerals, and healthy fats. One of the minerals found in salmon is sodium, which can be beneficial in the right amounts. Although too much sodium can be detrimental to health, the amount found in salmon is relatively low. A 3-ounce serving of cooked salmon contains approximately 60 milligrams of sodium, which is only 2.5% of the daily value. This means that even if you eat a lot of salmon, it is unlikely to contribute to an unhealthy sodium intake. In comparison, other types of fish, such as canned tuna, can contain up to 200 milligrams of sodium per 3-ounce serving. Salmon is also a good source of potassium, which can help to counteract the effects of sodium. Potassium helps to reduce blood pressure and keeps fluids balanced in the body. A 3-ounce serving of cooked salmon contains approximately 330 milligrams of potassium. Overall, salmon is an excellent source of lean protein and an array of vitamins and minerals. It is low in sodium and a great source of potassium, making it a healthy choice for those watching their sodium intake. It is also a great way to get your daily dose of omega-3 fatty acids, which are beneficial for heart health.

Tuna: Tuna is a type of fish that is high in protein and low in fat. It is a popular choice for many people who are looking for a healthy and delicious meal option. Tuna is also known for its high sodium content. Tuna contains a significant amount of sodium. A 3-ounce serving of canned tuna contains about 220 milligrams of sodium, which is about 10 percent of the recommended daily value for adults. This amount of sodium puts tuna at the high end of the average range for seafood. However, the sodium content of tuna can vary greatly depending on how it is prepared and packaged. For example, canned tuna packed in oil will have more sodium than tuna packed in water. Additionally, tuna prepared with added salt or other seasonings will have higher sodium levels than tuna that is simply cooked. Although tuna is high in sodium, that doesn't mean you have to avoid it. The key is to choose the right type of tuna and to watch your portion size. For example, opt for tuna packed in water instead of oil, and limit your intake to 3 ounces per day. Tuna is a healthy and delicious option that can be enjoyed in moderation. Just be sure to watch your sodium intake and opt for the lower sodium versions when possible.

Mackerel: Sodium is an essential nutrient found in many foods, including mackerel. Mackerel is a type of oily fish that is high in protein and Omega-3 fatty acids. It is also a good source of B vitamins, phosphorus, magnesium, and selenium. It is an excellent choice for those looking to increase their intake of healthy omega-3 fatty acids. In addition to its health benefits, mackerel is also a good source of sodium. A 3-ounce serving of cooked mackerel contains about 473 milligrams (mg) of sodium, which is about 20% of the daily recommended value for adults. This is equivalent to about 2.5 teaspoons of table salt. It is important to note that the sodium content of mackerel can vary depending on how it is prepared and cooked. For instance, canned mackerel may contain more sodium than fresh mackerel, as salt is often added during the canning process. Eating too much sodium can lead to high blood pressure and an increased risk of stroke and heart attack. Therefore, it is important to limit sodium intake to no more than 2,300 mg per day. To reduce the sodium content of mackerel, try grilling or baking it without adding extra salt. If you choose to purchase canned mackerel, opt for a variety labelled as "low sodium" or "no salt added." Additionally, make sure to rinse canned fish with water before using it in recipes. In conclusion, mackerel is a healthy and nutritious food that is high in protein and omega-3 fatty acids. It is a good source of sodium, but it is important to be mindful of how much sodium is in the fish. Try to limit sodium intake to no more than 2,300 mg per day and opt for fresh or low-sodium canned mackerel when possible.

Oysters: Sodium is also found naturally in a variety of foods, including oysters. Oysters are a type of shellfish that is high in minerals, including sodium. A single medium-sized oyster contains 13 mg of sodium, which is about 1% of the daily recommended intake for adults. This amount of sodium is considered low, making oysters a good choice for those who need to watch their sodium intake. In addition to providing a small amount of sodium, oysters are also an excellent source of other important minerals, such as zinc, iron, and selenium. They are also a good source of protein, which is important for muscle and bone health. Oysters are a great way to get the important minerals and nutrients your body needs, while keeping your sodium intake in check. Eating a variety of other low-sodium foods is also important for maintaining a healthy sodium balance. Some other low-sodium foods include fresh fruits and vegetables, nuts, legumes, and whole grains. Overall, oysters are a great source of sodium, as well as other essential minerals and nutrients. Eating a variety of low-sodium foods can help you maintain a healthy sodium balance and keep your body functioning properly.

Shrimp: Shrimp is a popular seafood choice that is enjoyed around the world. It is a great source of lean protein, vitamins and minerals, and omega-3 fatty acids. However, there is one nutrient that is often overlooked when it comes to shrimp – sodium. Sodium is an essential mineral that is necessary for the body to function properly. It helps regulate blood pressure, maintain fluid balance, and transmit nerve signals. The daily recommended intake for adults is about 2,300mg. While shrimp contains relatively low amounts of sodium, it can still be a significant contributor to the daily total. A 3-ounce serving of boiled shrimp contains approximately 130mg of sodium. This may not seem like much, but it adds up quickly when shrimp is eaten multiple times a week. It is important to be aware of how much sodium is in the shrimp and to take that into account when planning meals. In addition to the sodium content, shrimp also contains other substances that can have an effect on blood pressure. These substances include potassium, magnesium, and calcium. Potassium and magnesium help to balance out the effects of sodium, while calcium helps to reduce water retention. All of these substances are important for maintaining healthy blood pressure levels. When choosing shrimp, it is important to look for wild-caught varieties. Wild-caught shrimp tends to be lower in sodium than farmed shrimp, as farmed shrimp is often injected with a sodium solution to preserve it. It is also important to watch out for added sodium in sauces, marinades, and other toppings. Overall, shrimp can be an excellent source of lean protein and other essential nutrients. However, it is important to be aware of the sodium content and take steps to limit the amount of sodium consumed. Eating a variety of other low-sodium foods, such as fresh fruits and vegetables, can help to keep the overall sodium intake in check.

Cheese: Sodium is a mineral found in many foods, including cheese. It is an essential part of a healthy diet and is necessary for maintaining normal blood pressure and fluid balance. The amount of sodium in cheese varies greatly depending on the type of cheese, its age, and the processing method used. Cheeses that are made with raw milk contain the highest levels of sodium, while those made with pasteurized milk have lower levels. In general, fresh cheeses such as ricotta, cottage cheese, and cream cheese have the highest sodium content. Hard cheeses such as cheddar, Swiss, and Gouda have the lowest sodium content. Processed cheese products such as slices, spreads, and processed cheese foods have some of the highest sodium levels. These products often contain a variety of additives, preservatives, and sodium nitrate, a preservative and flavour enhancer, which can increase the sodium content of the cheese significantly. It is important to pay attention to the sodium levels in cheese when making dietary decisions. The American Heart Association recommends that adults limit their sodium intake to 2,300 milligrams per day, or 1,500 milligrams if you are 51 or older, African American, or have high blood pressure, diabetes, or chronic kidney disease. Cheese can be an important part of a healthy diet, but it is important to be aware of the sodium content in the type of cheese you choose. Limiting processed cheese products and opting for fresh cheeses can help you reduce your sodium intake.

Butter: Sodium is found in many foods, including butter. While butter is a source of beneficial nutrients, it can also be high in sodium, depending on the type and brand. Butter is made from cream that has been churned until it forms a solid. Most butter contains at least 80% fat, with the remainder being made up of water, proteins, and minerals, including sodium. Depending on the product, the amount of sodium can range from 10 to 120 milligrams per tablespoon. Unsalted butter, also known as sweet cream butter, is the most common type of butter and contains the least amount of sodium. It is usually made from pasteurized cream and is free from added salt. The amount of sodium in unsalted butter is typically around 10 milligrams per tablespoon. Salted butter, on the other hand, is made from cream that has been churned with added salt. This type of butter contains more sodium, typically around 120 milligrams per tablespoon. It is often used in baking or cooking as the added salt enhances the flavour of the dish. When it comes to sodium, there are some things to consider. Too much sodium can be harmful to your health, as it can increase your risk of developing high blood pressure, stroke, heart disease, and kidney disease. On the flip side, too little sodium can also be problematic, as it can lead to low blood pressure, cramps, and other issues. For most people, the amount of sodium in butter is not a major concern, as it is typically only a small portion of the total amount of sodium in their diet. However, if you are trying to reduce your sodium intake, it is important to check the nutrition facts label and compare products to find the one with the lowest sodium content. In conclusion, sodium is found in butter, but the amount varies depending on the type and brand. Unsalted butter is the best choice if you are looking to reduce your sodium intake. However, it is important to remember that too much or too little sodium can be harmful to your health, so it is important to find a balance that works for you.

Sulfur

Sulfur is an essential mineral found in many foods. It is a vital component of proteins and is necessary for the body to form amino acids. It is also important for a healthy immune system, as well as for skin, hair, and nail health. Sulfur is found in a variety of foods, including fish, eggs, dairy products, legumes, nuts, and grains. It can also be found in some fruits and vegetables, such as onions and garlic. Sulfur is important for the body because it helps create essential amino acids, which are needed for the formation of proteins. It also plays a role in the production of important enzymes that help break down food and absorb nutrients. It is also important for metabolic processes, such as digestion and energy production. In addition to its role in the body, sulfur is also important for the environment. It helps reduce the amount of pollutants in the air, as well as helps to neutralize acid rain. When it comes to your diet, you should aim to get about 700-800 milligrams of sulfur per day. This can be easily achieved by eating a balanced diet that includes a variety of foods from the different food groups. In summary, sulfur is an essential mineral found in many foods. It is important for the body because it helps create essential amino acids and is necessary for a healthy immune system. It is also important for metabolic processes, such as digestion and energy production. You should aim to get about 700-800 milligrams of sulfur per day by eating a balanced diet.

Sulfur is an essential mineral found in many foods and is important for optimal health and wellbeing. It is a vital component of amino acids, proteins, and enzymes that assist in many important body processes. Sulfur also helps to protect cells and tissues from oxidative damage, as it acts as an antioxidant, and helps to detoxify the body. Sulfur plays an important role in the health of bones, joints, cartilage, and connective tissues. It helps to keep these structures lubricated, flexible, and strong. As we age, our bodies produce less sulfur, so it is important to include sulfur-rich foods in our diets. Sulfur helps to regulate the body's pH levels, which helps to maintain a healthy balance of acidity and alkalinity. It also helps to transport oxygen and nutrients to the cells, as well as to remove waste and toxins from the body. Sulfur also helps to reduce inflammation, which can help to relieve pain and discomfort.

Sulfur helps to reduce swelling and inflammation, which can help to improve joint pain, arthritis, and other inflammatory conditions. Sulfur is essential for the production of collagen, a protein that helps to keep skin looking young and healthy. It is also important for the production of keratin, a protein that helps to form hair, nails, and skin. Sulfur is also important for the production of certain hormones, such as insulin and glucagon. Insulin helps to regulate blood sugar levels, while glucagon helps to break down fats and proteins in the body. In conclusion, sulfur is an important mineral that plays an essential role in many important body processes. It helps to protect cells and tissues from oxidative damage, regulate pH levels, reduce inflammation, and produce collagen, keratin, and hormones. Therefore, it is important to include sulfur-rich foods in our diets to ensure optimal health and wellbeing.

Food sources

Sulfur is an important element found in many foods.

Turkey: Turkey is a source of dietary sulfur, containing both organic and inorganic forms. The organic forms of sulfur, like cysteine and methionine, are found in the protein portion of the turkey. Inorganic sulfur is found in the form of sulphates and sulphites, which are added to some processed foods for flavour and colour. Sulfur found in turkey plays a role in many of its nutritional benefits. It helps the body to absorb important minerals, like iron and zinc, which are essential for good health. Sulfur also helps to break down proteins and other complex molecules into simpler forms that can be used by the body. Sulfur can also be beneficial for preventing certain types of cancer. Studies have found that sulfur-containing foods, such as turkey, may help to reduce the risk of certain types of cancer, including colon, breast, and prostate cancer. The sulfur-containing compounds in turkey may also help to protect against heart disease by reducing levels of bad cholesterol in the body. For these reasons, it is important to include turkey, and other sulfur-rich foods, in your diet.

Beef: Sulfur is an essential element in the diet of beef cattle. It helps to build proteins, is used in the formation of essential amino acids, and is involved in the production of energy in cells. The amount of sulfur present in beef can vary depending on the diet of the animal, its age, and the breed of cattle. Generally, younger animals have higher levels of sulfur than older animals. Sulfur is important for the health and well-being of beef cattle. It plays a role in the metabolism of fats, carbohydrates, and proteins, as well as in the production of energy. It also helps to maintain proper mineral balance, acid-base balance, and muscle pH. In addition, sulfur is essential for the production of hormones, enzymes, and other compounds involved in growth and development. Sulfur is also involved in the synthesis of nucleic acids, fatty acids, and glucose. High levels of sulfur in beef can lead to an unpleasant taste and odour, as well as a yellow or green discoloration. For this reason, it is important to monitor the sulfur content of beef and ensure that it meets the required standards. In general, beef should not contain more than 0.2% sulfur on a dry matter basis. Sulfur levels can be reduced through proper nutrition, such as adding sulfur-rich supplements or reducing the intake of sulfur-containing feeds. In conclusion, sulfur is an important element in the diet of beef cattle. It plays a role in the metabolism and production of energy, as well as in the synthesis of hormones and enzymes. High levels of sulfur can lead to an unpleasant taste and odour, so it is important to monitor the sulfur content of beef and ensure that it meets the required standards.

Chicken: Sulfur is an essential mineral that is found in chicken. It is a component of several proteins, including cysteine, methionine, and taurine. It is also found in the vitamins thiamine and biotin. Sulfur is important for many bodily functions, including energy production and cell health. Sulfur is present in chicken in the form of amino acids, particularly cysteine, methionine, and taurine. Cysteine is an amino acid that is used in the formation of proteins, while methionine is involved in many metabolic pathways and can be converted into cysteine. Taurine is an amino acid involved in fat metabolism and energy production. The sulfur content in chicken can vary depending on the breed of chicken as well as the feed they are eating. Generally, chickens raised on a diet of grain-based feed have higher levels of sulfur than those fed on grass or forage. The sulfur content of chicken can also vary depending on its age and the method of cooking. For example, boiling chicken reduces its sulfur content, while roasting increases it. The health benefits of sulfur in chicken include improved joint health, better digestion, and stronger bones and teeth. It is also thought to have anti-inflammatory properties and may reduce the risk of certain types of cancer. Overall, sulfur is an essential mineral for the body and is found in chicken.

Eggs: Sulfur is an important component of eggs. It is found in the yolk and albumen, or white of the egg. Sulfur is found in eggs in two forms – organic and inorganic. Organic sulfur is found in the egg yolk and is bound to proteins, fats, and carbohydrates. This form of sulfur is easily absorbed by the body and provides it with the essential nutrients it needs to function properly. Inorganic sulfur is found in the albumen, or white of the egg. This form of sulfur is not easily absorbed by the body, but it is still beneficial as it helps to maintain the egg's firmness and structure. The health benefits of sulfur in eggs are numerous. It helps to maintain healthy bones and teeth, as well as aiding in the formation of new cells and repairing damaged ones. Sulfur also helps to regulate blood sugar levels, reduce inflammation, and boost the immune system. Additionally, sulfur is important for the absorption of other essential vitamins and minerals, such as iron and calcium. Eggs are also a great source of other important vitamins and minerals. They are a good source of protein and healthy fats, as well as containing vitamins A, B, and E. Eggs are also a good source of iron, zinc, magnesium, and potassium. Eggs are a versatile food that can be incorporated into a variety of dishes. They can be boiled, scrambled, or used in baking. Eggs can also be added to salads, omelettes, and quiches. Eating eggs is a great way to get the essential vitamins and minerals your body needs. They are a good source of protein, healthy fats, and essential vitamins and minerals. They also contain sulfur, which is essential for the proper functioning of many bodily systems. Eating eggs regularly can help to keep you healthy and energized.

Fish: Sulfur is an important element in the fish's diet, as it plays several key roles in their health and development. In fish, sulfur is found in the form of amino acids, which are necessary for protein synthesis. Amino acids are also essential for muscle development and growth, as well as for maintaining healthy skin and scales. Additionally, sulfur helps regulate the pH balance of the fish's body, making it less susceptible to disease. Sulfur is also important for the production of energy in the fish. It is necessary for the transport of oxygen and the conversion of nutrients into energy. Furthermore, sulfur helps to regulate the osmotic balance within the fish, allowing them to maintain their internal environment. Finally, sulfur helps to protect the fish from oxidative damage, which can come from environmental pollutants and other toxins. When considering the dietary needs of your fish, it is important to make sure that they are receiving adequate amounts of sulfur. In general, a good source of sulfur is found in the form of fish meal, which is a combination of fish proteins, oils, and other nutrients. Additionally, some commercial fish foods contain additional sulfur, usually in the form of alfalfa meal or kelp powder. You can also supplement your fish's diet with other sources of sulfur, such as dried seaweed, eggs, and shrimp. In order to ensure that your fish are receiving enough sulfur, it is important to monitor their diet and supplement it as necessary. If you find that your fish are not receiving enough sulfur, you can supplement their diet with a sulfur-rich food. Additionally, it is important to test your fish's water for sulfur levels, as too much or too little sulfur can be harmful to their health. Overall, sulfur is an essential element in the health and development of fish. It is important to make sure that your fish are receiving adequate amounts of sulfur in their diet, as this will help them to stay healthy and active. With proper monitoring and supplementation, you can ensure that your fish receive the sulfur they need to remain healthy and happy.

Nuts: Sulfur is found naturally in many foods, including nuts. Almonds, cashews, and peanuts are all high in sulfur. One ounce of almonds contains 335 milligrams of sulfur, while one ounce of cashews contains 253 milligrams, and one ounce of peanuts contains 247 milligrams. Other nuts, such as walnuts and pistachios, also contain sulfur, though not in as high of concentrations. The sulfur found in nuts is beneficial to the body and helps to support the body's natural detoxification processes. Sulfur helps to rid the body of toxins, which can help to improve overall health. Nuts are a great source of healthy fats, protein, and fibre, and are a great snack to have on hand for when hunger strikes. Eating them in moderation can help to ensure that you're getting enough sulfur in your diet. In addition to nuts, sulfur can also be found in other foods such as eggs, fish, dairy, legumes, and some vegetables. Eating a balanced diet that includes a variety of these foods is the best way to ensure that you're getting enough sulfur in your diet. Overall, nuts are a great source of sulfur, and can be a healthy and delicious snack when eaten in moderation. Eating a variety of foods that contain sulfur can help to ensure that your body is getting all the sulfur it needs to stay healthy.

Seeds: The sulfur in seeds helps to form proteins, which are necessary for the growth and development of the plant. These proteins can be found in the cell walls of the seed, as well as in the proteins that are found in the seed's endosperm. The sulfur found in the endosperm is known as the "storage form" of sulfur, and it is used by the plant for growth and development. Sulfur also plays an important role in the formation of vitamins and enzymes. It helps to break down carbohydrates, proteins and fats, and is necessary for the production of vitamins such as thiamine, riboflavin and niacin. It also helps to break down fats and helps to form enzymes that are important for the production of energy. Sulfur is also important for the formation of certain hormones, such as auxins and gibberellins. These hormones play an important role in the growth and development of the plant, and the sulfur in the seed helps to form these hormones. Sulfur is also necessary for the formation of chlorophyll, which helps the plant to absorb energy from the sun. Without this element, the plant would not be able to produce the energy it needs to grow and develop. In summary, sulfur is an important element in the formation of proteins, vitamins and enzymes in plants. It is also necessary for the formation of certain hormones and for the absorption of energy from the sun. Seeds are a major source of sulfur and are necessary for healthy growth and development of the plant.

Legumes: Sulfur is an essential mineral nutrient found in legumes, such as beans, peas, and lentils, that is essential for plant growth, health, and overall nutrition. It is a component of proteins, enzymes, vitamins, and other important molecules, and is necessary for the synthesis of important amino acids. Sulfur is found in both the soil and air and is a key component of the photosynthesis process. In legumes, sulfur plays an important role in the production of proteins, enzymes, vitamins, and other important molecules. It is essential for the synthesis of some of the essential amino acids, such as methionine and cysteine, and is important for the formation of other important molecules, such as thiamine, riboflavin, and biotin. Sulfur also plays a role in the production of certain vitamins, including vitamin B1, B2, and B6. Sulfur helps to improve the taste and texture of legumes and can also increase their nutritional value. It aids in the breakdown of proteins and carbohydrates and helps to regulate the acidity of the soil. Sulfur also helps to promote root growth and helps to increase the availability of certain minerals and elements, such as magnesium, calcium, and iron. In legumes, sulfur is available in the form of sulphates, which are compounds that contain the element sulfur. These compounds can be found naturally in legumes, or they can be added to the soil or water. Sulphates are also available as supplements, but it is important to read the label and make sure that the product contains the right amount of sulfur for the particular legume crop. In order to ensure that legumes are getting the adequate amount of sulfur, it is important to monitor the pH of the soil, as sulfur is more available in soils with higher pH levels. In addition, sulfur can be added to the soil in the form of fertilizers and compost. Overall, sulfur is an important mineral nutrient found in legumes, and it is essential for plant growth, health, and overall nutrition. It is a key component of proteins, enzymes, vitamins, and other important molecules, and is necessary for the synthesis of some of the essential amino acids. Sulfur is also important for improving the taste and texture of legumes, and for promoting root growth and increasing the availability of certain minerals and elements. To ensure that legumes are getting the adequate amount of sulfur, it is important to monitor the pH of the soil, as well as to add sulfur to the soil in the form of fertilizers and compost.

Allium Vegetables: Sulfur is an essential element for plant growth and development, and it's also a key component in the flavour and aroma of many vegetables, including allium vegetables such as onions, garlic, leeks, and scallions. Allium vegetables contain sulfur-containing compounds called thiosulfates, which are responsible for the characteristic smell and flavour of these veggies. Thiosulfates are formed when an enzyme called alliinase breaks down the amino acid alliin, which is found in allium vegetables. When the enzymes break down alliin, they create thiosulfates that are responsible for the pungent smell and flavour associated with these vegetables. Thiosulfates are also believed to have health benefits, as they have been shown to have antimicrobial and anti-inflammatory properties. In addition to thiosulfates, allium vegetables also contain sulfur-containing compounds called sulfoxides. These compounds are responsible for the sharp, intense flavour of allium vegetables, as well as their pungent aroma. Sulfoxides are thought to have a positive effect on the cardiovascular system, as well as anti-cancer properties. When cooking allium vegetables, it's important to remember that the sulfur compounds are released when the vegetables are cut, chopped, or crushed. Cooking methods such as boiling, steaming, and baking can reduce the amount of sulfur compounds released, while sautéing and frying can increase the amount. Overall, sulfur is an important component of allium vegetables, contributing to both their flavour and aroma. The sulfur-containing compounds in allium vegetables are believed to have health benefits, and the amount of sulfur released when cooking can be affected by the cooking method used.

Cruciferous Vegetables: Sulfur is an important element that plays a vital role in many biological processes. It is a component of proteins, enzymes, hormones, vitamins, and even DNA. Cruciferous vegetables such as cabbage, Brussels sprouts, broccoli, and cauliflower are some of the best sources of sulfur. Sulfur is essential for the production of essential amino acids. These amino acids are the building blocks of proteins, which are essential for growth and development. Without sulfur, proteins cannot be properly constructed and synthesized, which can lead to a number of health issues. Sulfur also helps to regulate the body's metabolism. It helps to break down carbohydrates, fat, and protein into energy. It also helps the body to absorb vitamins and minerals and assists in the production of hormones such as insulin and glucagon. Sulfur also plays a role in detoxification. It helps the body to flush out toxins and waste products, which can help to prevent disease. Sulfur also helps to reduce inflammation and can be beneficial for skin conditions such as psoriasis and eczema. Cruciferous vegetables are some of the best sources of sulfur. They are high in dietary fibre, vitamins, minerals and antioxidants, and are also a good source of protein and iron. Eating cruciferous vegetables on a regular basis can help to ensure that the body gets all the sulfur it needs. In conclusion, sulfur is an important element that plays an important role in many biological processes. Cruciferous vegetables such as cabbage, Brussels sprouts, broccoli, and cauliflower are some of the best sources of sulfur. Eating cruciferous vegetables on a regular basis can help to ensure that the body gets all the sulfur it needs.

TRACE MINERALS

Trace minerals are essential for human health and for the functioning of all living organisms. They are vital for a wide range of bodily processes and are present in extremely small amounts in the human body. Trace minerals are found in small amounts in soil, water, and food, and although they are only needed in small amounts, they are essential for proper health and functioning. Trace minerals are a group of minerals that are essential for the functioning of the body. They are necessary for the formation and maintenance of bones, teeth, and muscles, and they are involved in many other biochemical processes. They are also needed for the proper functioning of the immune system, reproduction, and growth. Trace minerals are divided into two categories: microminerals and microminerals. Microminerals are needed in larger amounts and include calcium, phosphorus, magnesium, sodium, potassium, and chloride. Microminerals are needed in smaller amounts and include iron, zinc, copper, manganese, selenium, iodine, chromium, molybdenum, and fluoride. The human body needs trace minerals for many different functions. They are essential for the formation and maintenance of bones, teeth, and muscles, and they are involved in many other biochemical processes. They are needed for the proper functioning of the immune system, reproduction, and growth. They also help to regulate heartbeat, blood pressure, and fluid balance. Trace minerals are also important for proper nerve and brain function, digestion, and metabolism. The body obtains trace minerals through food and water. The best sources of trace minerals are plant-based foods such as fruits, vegetables, nuts, seeds, and grains. Animal-based foods such as meat, fish, dairy, and eggs also contain trace minerals but in lower amounts. It is important to get a variety of foods to ensure you get enough trace minerals. Some processed foods may also contain trace minerals, but it is important to check the label to make sure the food contains the minerals your body needs. In conclusion, trace minerals are essential for human health and for the functioning of all living organisms. They are needed in small amounts, but they are essential for proper health and functioning. Trace minerals are divided into two categories: microminerals and microminerals. They can be obtained through a variety of foods, and it is important to get a variety of foods to ensure you get enough trace minerals.

Trace minerals are essential nutrients that are needed in very small amounts by the human body to keep it functioning properly. They are involved in the formation of hormones, enzymes, and other important molecules, and they are also important for maintaining electrolyte balance and hydration. Trace minerals are also crucial for healthy bones, teeth, and skin. Trace minerals play a key role in the body's metabolism and energy production. They help convert food into energy, as well as aiding in the formation of red blood cells, which are essential for oxygen transport. In addition, trace minerals help regulate blood pressure and the pH balance in the body. They also help to keep the immune system functioning at its best. Trace minerals are important for the formation of connective tissue, which is necessary for the proper functioning of the body's organs. They also help to keep the nervous system functioning at its best, and they play a role in muscle contraction. Trace minerals are even involved in the production of neurotransmitters, which are responsible for carrying messages throughout the body. Lastly, trace minerals are important for healthy hair, nails, and skin. They help to keep these areas of the body strong and healthy, and they also help to protect them from damage and disease. Overall, trace minerals are important for the body's overall health and well-being. They are involved in a variety of processes, and they are essential for the body to function properly. For these reasons, it is important to make sure that you are getting enough trace minerals in your diet. Foods that are rich in trace minerals include seafood, seaweed, nuts, seeds, and some fruits and vegetables. You can also take a supplement to make sure you are getting enough trace minerals.

Trace minerals are essential nutrients required in the human body in small amounts. They are found in a variety of foods, including grains, vegetables, fruits, dairy products, and meats. Trace minerals are important for many bodily functions, including energy production, hormone production, and immune system function. The number of trace minerals varies depending on which source you consult. According to the National Institutes of Health, there are a total of 15 trace minerals that are considered essential for health.

Iron

Iron is an essential nutrient that is found in food and is necessary for human health. It is an important part of our diet and helps to keep us healthy by allowing the body to use oxygen, helping the immune system fight off infection, and providing energy for the body. Iron comes in two forms, heme and non-heme. Heme iron is found in animal sources, like red meat and fish, and is easily absorbed by the body. Non-heme iron is found in plant sources, like beans and dark leafy greens, and is less easily absorbed. The recommended daily intake of iron for adults is 8 to 18 mg per day. Women of childbearing age, pregnant women, and athletes need even more iron to stay healthy. The daily recommended intake of iron for children and teenagers ranges from 10 to 15 mg per day. Iron deficiency is a common problem, especially among women of childbearing age and pregnant women. Iron deficiency can cause anemia, which is a condition that makes people feel tired and weak. It can also cause poor concentration, fatigue, and other health problems. Getting enough iron in your diet is important for maintaining good health. Eating a balanced diet with a variety of foods is the best way to get enough iron. Good sources of heme iron include red meat, fish, poultry, and shellfish. Plant sources of non-heme iron include beans, dark leafy greens, nuts, and fortified cereals. Iron supplements are also available and can help people who are deficient in iron. However, it is important to talk to a doctor before taking any supplements, as too much iron can be harmful. In conclusion, iron is an essential nutrient that is found in food and is necessary for human health. Eating a balanced diet with a variety of foods is the best way to get enough iron. Iron supplements are also available to help people who are deficient in iron, but it is important to talk to a doctor before taking any supplements.

Zinc

Zinc is an essential nutrient found in many foods. It is an important component of many enzymes, proteins, and hormones that play a crucial role in numerous bodily processes. Zinc is also important for a healthy immune system, the production of red blood cells, wound healing, and the maintenance of vision and smell. Zinc is found naturally in a variety of foods, including meat, poultry, seafood, dairy products, nuts, legumes, and whole grains. Oysters are one of the richest sources of zinc, providing up to 74 mg per 3-ounce serving. Other good sources include beef, pork, and fortified breakfast cereals. Zinc is an essential trace mineral that is important for a wide range of bodily functions, including growth and development, DNA synthesis, and immune system function. It is also involved in wound healing and the production of new cells. Zinc deficiency can lead to a variety of health issues, such as impaired cognitive development, weakened immune system, and increased risk of infection. The Recommended Dietary Allowance (RDA) for zinc is 8 mg per day for adults. However, pregnant women and breastfeeding mothers should aim for 11 and 12 mg per day, respectively. For children, the RDA ranges from 3 mg to 8 mg per day, depending on age. It is important to note that zinc absorption can be reduced if consumed with certain foods or drinks such as fibre, calcium, or phytates. For this reason, it is important to get zinc from a variety of sources and to spread out consumption throughout the day. Including zinc-rich foods in your diet is an important way to ensure your body is getting the zinc it needs. Eating a balanced diet that includes a variety of zinc-rich foods is the best way to ensure your body is getting the essential nutrients it needs for optimal health.

Copper

Copper is an essential trace mineral found in many foods. It plays an important role in human health, as it is necessary for energy production, nerve transmission, and the absorption of iron. Copper also helps maintain healthy bones and is important for the formation of blood vessels and muscle tissue. Copper is found in many foods, such as organ meats, seafood, nuts, legumes, and whole grains. It is also present in fruits, vegetables, and dairy products. Copper can be found in fortified foods, such as breakfast cereals, and in some plant-based foods, such as soybeans and tempeh. The human body does not produce copper, so it is important to get enough of it from dietary sources. The recommended daily amount for adults is between 900 and 1,200 mcg per day. It is important to note that consuming too much copper can have negative effects on health, so it is important to find a balance in the diet. When preparing food, it is important to consider how copper affects food. Copper can react with certain ingredients and cause discoloration, off-flavours, or a metallic taste. To reduce the risk of this occurring, it is important to use copper cookware and utensils that are lined with a non-reactive material, such as stainless steel, titanium, or enamel. Copper is an essential mineral that should be included in the diet to ensure health and optimal functioning. Although it is important to get enough copper from dietary sources, it is also important to take precautions when cooking with copper to avoid any negative reactions. By finding a balance between dietary sources and proper cooking techniques, you can ensure that you are getting the right amount of copper in your diet.

Selenium

Selenium is an important trace element found in food that plays a vital role in our health. It is an essential mineral that is required in small amounts for the proper functioning of the human body. In particular, it is necessary for the proper functioning of the immune system, thyroid gland, and reproductive organs. Selenium is found naturally in some foods, especially those that come from animal sources such as fish, poultry, and eggs. It is also found in nuts, grains, and certain vegetables. In addition, some types of soil are known to have high levels of selenium, which can be absorbed through crops grown in those soils. The daily recommended intake of selenium for adults is 55 mcg. However, it is important to get enough selenium in your diet as it is essential for many bodily processes. For instance, it helps to protect cells from damage due to oxidative stress, helps to regulate the thyroid hormone, and helps to produce antioxidant enzymes that can protect against disease. In addition, selenium helps to regulate the immune system, which is important for fighting off infections and diseases. It can also help to improve cognitive functioning and reduce the risk of certain types of cancer. For those who are unable to get enough selenium through their diet, it is possible to supplement with selenium-rich foods or take a selenium supplement. Selenium supplements are available in tablet, capsule, or liquid forms, and should be taken according to the instructions on the label. Overall, selenium is an important trace element that is necessary for the proper functioning of the human body. It is important to get enough of this mineral through your diet or through supplementation if necessary.

Iodine

Iodine is an essential mineral that plays an important role in human health. It is a component of thyroid hormones, which help regulate your metabolism, energy levels, and body temperature. While the body doesn't make iodine naturally, it can be found in a variety of foods, including iodized salt, seafood, seaweed, milk, yogurt, eggs, and bread. Iodine is an important nutrient in the diet, as it helps the body produce thyroid hormones, which are necessary for growth, development, and metabolism. Iodine is also important for proper functioning of the immune system, as well as the prevention of certain diseases, such as goitre and cretinism. The recommended dietary allowance (RDA) of iodine is 150 mcg per day for adults. However, pregnant and breastfeeding women should aim for higher levels of iodine, as the fetus or baby will also need iodine. Iodized salt is one of the most common sources of iodine in the diet. It is a salt that has been fortified with iodine and is widely available in most grocery stores. While iodized salt is a good source of iodine, it is important to be mindful of the amount you consume, as too much salt can increase your risk of high blood pressure and other health problems. Seafood is another great source of iodine, as most fish and shellfish contain high levels of the mineral. For example, a 3 ounce serving of cod provides 99 mcg of iodine, while a 3 ounce serving of shrimp provides 35 mcg. Other seafood sources of iodine include salmon, tuna, and oysters. Seaweed is also a good source of iodine, especially varieties such as kelp and nori. A 1/4 cup of dried seaweed can provide up to 2,984 mcg of iodine. In comparison, a 3 ounce serving of cod provides 99 mcg. Milk, yogurt, and eggs are also good sources of iodine, as they are often enriched with the mineral. A 1 cup serving of milk can provide 56 mcg of iodine, while a 1/2 cup of yogurt can provide up to 75 mcg. As for eggs, a large egg can provide up to 24 mcg of iodine. Finally, many breads are fortified with iodine, so be sure to check the label for the iodine content. A 2 slice serving of whole wheat bread can provide up to 45 mcg of iodine. In conclusion, iodine is an essential mineral that plays an important role in human health. It can be found in a variety of foods, including iodized salt, seafood, seaweed, milk, yogurt, eggs, and bread. Eating a balanced diet with a variety of iodine-rich foods is the best way to ensure that you meet your daily iodine needs.

Cobalt

Cobalt is a trace element found in a variety of foods, including meats, seafood, dairy products, leafy green vegetables, and grains. While cobalt is an essential nutrient, its presence in food is often quite low and it's not a nutrient that many people think about. However, it plays an important role in healthy nutrition, as it helps the body absorb and utilize essential vitamins and minerals. Cobalt is an essential component of vitamin B12, which is critical for energy metabolism, red blood cell production, and neurological development. It is also necessary for the formation of haemoglobin, which transports oxygen in the blood. Without adequate cobalt, the body can't properly utilize vitamin B12 or absorb other important nutrients such as iron, zinc, and magnesium. Cobalt can be found in a variety of animal-based foods, including beef, pork, lamb, chicken, fish, and shellfish. Dairy products, such as cheese and yogurt, are also sources of cobalt. Plant-based sources include legumes, nuts, and some grains, such as oats and barley. Leafy green vegetables, such as spinach and kale, and some fruits, such as raspberries and blackberries, are also good sources of cobalt. The recommended daily intake of cobalt is 2-3 micrograms for adults. Pregnant and breastfeeding women should increase their intake to 4-5 micrograms per day. While cobalt is found in a variety of foods, deficiencies can occur if the diet is lacking in certain nutrients, such as vitamin B12, or if the body has difficulty absorbing cobalt. Symptoms of cobalt deficiency include anemia, fatigue, and poor growth. In general, a balanced diet that includes a variety of foods should provide all the cobalt your body needs. However, if you're concerned about your cobalt intake, talk to your doctor or dietitian. They may suggest a supplement or other dietary changes to ensure that you are meeting your needs.

Manganese

Manganese is a trace mineral found in small amounts in the human body. It is essential for many body functions and plays a key role in metabolism, bone health, and nerve and muscle function. While it is not considered an essential nutrient, it is still important for the body to get enough of it. Manganese can be found in many foods, such as nuts, beans, grains, and leafy green vegetables. Manganese plays a role in the formation of connective tissue, cartilage, and bones, and is also necessary for the formation of enzymes that break down fats, carbohydrates, and proteins. It helps to regulate blood sugar levels and is a component of many enzymes involved in energy production and antioxidant defence. Manganese is also essential for the proper functioning of the nervous system and for the formation of neurotransmitters. Manganese is found in a wide variety of foods, including nuts and seeds, beans, oats, wheat germ, and some fruits and vegetables. It is also found in some seafood, such as oysters, mussels, and crabs. Additionally, some herbs and spices, such as coriander, thyme, and nutmeg, also contain manganese. Manganese deficiency is rare, but can occur in people with certain medical conditions, such as Crohn's disease, celiac disease, and anorexia nervosa. Symptoms of manganese deficiency include fatigue, poor concentration, irritability, and muscle weakness. A balanced diet that includes a variety of foods from the major food groups is the best way to ensure adequate intake of manganese. There is no recommended daily allowance of manganese established by the Food and Nutrition Board, but the Institute of Medicine recommends that adult men and women consume 2.3 milligrams and 1.8 milligrams of manganese, respectively, per day. Eating a variety of foods that contain manganese can help ensure that one obtains the recommended daily allowance of this important mineral.

Chromium

Chromium is an essential trace mineral that plays a vital role in the metabolism of carbohydrates, fats, and proteins. It is found in many foods, including whole grains, meats, cheeses, fruits, vegetables, and legumes. Chromium is also found in some dietary supplements. The human body needs chromium to process glucose, which is the body's primary source of energy. Chromium helps to move glucose from the bloodstream into the cells, where it can be used as fuel. Without it, glucose can remain in the bloodstream, leading to elevated blood sugar levels. Chromium also helps to improve insulin sensitivity, which can help to regulate blood sugar levels. Chromium is also important for maintaining healthy cholesterol levels. It helps to prevent the build-up of bad cholesterol, which can lead to heart disease. Chromium also helps to boost HDL (good) cholesterol, which helps to protect against heart disease. Chromium is important for the metabolism of proteins, fats, and carbohydrates, and it helps with healthy weight management. Chromium helps to convert carbohydrates into energy and helps to regulate appetite. It also helps to break down lipids (fats) and proteins, which are important for cell growth and repair. In addition to its role in metabolism, chromium is also important for proper brain and nerve function. It helps to improve memory and concentration, and it can help to reduce depression and anxiety. Most people get enough chromium from their diet, but some people may be deficient in chromium. This includes people who have certain medical conditions, such as diabetes, or those taking certain medications. People who are at risk of chromium deficiency may want to consider taking a chromium supplement to ensure they are getting enough of the mineral. Chromium is found in many foods, including whole grains, meats, cheeses, fruits, vegetables, and legumes. It is also found in some dietary supplements. To ensure you are getting enough chromium, it is important to eat a well-balanced diet that includes a variety of these foods.

Molybdenum

Molybdenum is a trace mineral found in a variety of foods and is essential for human nutrition. It is found in some of the most common food sources including whole grain cereals, legumes, dairy products, leafy green vegetables, nuts, and organ meats. Molybdenum is an important component of enzymes and helps to regulate the metabolism of iron, sulfur, and nitrogen in the body. The recommended daily allowance (RDA) of molybdenum is 45 micrograms (mcg) for adults. This amount is increased to 75 mcg for pregnant women, as they require more of the mineral to meet their needs. Molybdenum plays a key role in several metabolic pathways. It helps to convert nitrates into nitrites, and also aids in the metabolism of carbohydrates, amino acids, and lipids. It also plays a role in the metabolism of vitamin B12 and helps to reduce the risk of anemia and other blood-related disorders. In addition to its metabolic role, molybdenum is also important for the formation of collagen, which is essential for healthy bones, teeth, and gums. It also helps to protect against a variety of cancers, including liver and colorectal cancer. Molybdenum is most commonly found in plant-based foods such as legumes, whole grains, nuts, and leafy green vegetables. It is also found in animal foods such as organ meats, dairy products, and fish. Some of the highest sources of molybdenum include lentils, kidney beans, chickpeas, oats, and spinach. When it comes to supplements, molybdenum is available in a variety of forms including tablets, capsules, and liquids. Supplements should only be taken under the supervision of a healthcare professional, as it is possible to overdose on the mineral. In conclusion, molybdenum is an important trace mineral that plays a key role in several metabolic pathways. It is found in foods such as legumes, whole grains, nuts, leafy green vegetables, and animal sources. It is also available in supplement form but should only be taken under the supervision of a healthcare professional.

Vanadium

Vanadium is a trace element found in small amounts in some foods. It is an essential mineral that plays an important role in metabolism, but most people don't get enough of it in their diets. Vanadium is found in many foods, including fruits, vegetables, legumes, grains, and nuts. It is also found in some fish, such as salmon and tuna. Vanadium is essential for healthy bones and teeth, as well as for proper growth and development. It also helps to regulate the body's insulin levels, which is important for controlling blood sugar levels. Vanadium also helps to support the immune system and may even have anti-cancer properties. Vanadium is found in a variety of foods, but the highest concentrations are found in mushrooms, shellfish, kidney beans, and grains, such as oats and wheat germ. It is also found in spinach and other dark green leafy vegetables. Nuts, such as almonds and Brazil nuts, are also good sources of vanadium. The recommended daily allowance for vanadium is about 5-15 mcg for adults. However, it is very difficult to get enough vanadium from food sources alone, so it is often recommended to take a supplement to meet your needs. In general, vanadium is an important mineral that plays an essential role in the body. It helps to regulate blood sugar levels, supports the immune system, and may even have anti-cancer properties. While it can be found in a variety of foods, it is often difficult to get enough vanadium from food sources alone, so it may be necessary to take a supplement in order to meet your recommended daily allowance.

Boron

Boron is an essential trace mineral found in food that plays an important role in maintaining the health of humans and animals. It is found in all parts of the plant, including the leaves, stems, roots, fruits, and seeds. In humans, boron is essential for the normal functioning of the body, including the metabolism of carbohydrates, proteins, and fats, as well as the maintenance of bone and joint health. Boron is found in a wide variety of foods, including fruits, vegetables, nuts, grains, meats, and dairy products. Fruits and vegetables are particularly rich sources of boron, with apples, pears, grapes, avocados, and apricots being some of the best sources. Nuts and seeds, such as almonds, walnuts, and peanuts, are also good sources of boron. Grains, including whole wheat, oats, and rice, are also good sources of boron, as are legumes, such as beans, lentils, and peas. Meats, such as beef, pork, and chicken, also contain small amounts of boron. Dairy products, including milk, yogurt, and cheese, are also good sources of boron. Boron is an important mineral for overall health, as it helps to maintain healthy bones and joints, as well as aiding in the metabolism of carbohydrates, proteins, and fats. It also helps to regulate hormone levels and can help to reduce inflammation and improve cognitive performance. In addition, boron can help to reduce the risk of certain types of cancer, as well as helping to protect against osteoporosis. For adults, the recommended daily allowance of boron is 3 to 4 milligrams. This can easily be obtained through a healthy diet that includes a variety of fruits, vegetables, nuts, grains, meats, and dairy products. For those who are unable to obtain enough boron through their diet, supplementation may be necessary. However, it is always best to consult with a healthcare professional before taking any supplements.

FIBRE

Fibre is an important component of a healthy diet, providing essential nutrition and helping to keep your digestive system running smoothly. Fibre is a type of carbohydrate that is not digested and absorbed by your body, but instead passes through your digestive system largely unchanged. Fibre can be found in a variety of different foods, including fruits, vegetables, whole grains, nuts, and legumes. It is also found in some processed foods, such as cereals and bran-based products. Fibre is categorized as either soluble or insoluble. Soluble fibre dissolves in water, forming a gel-like substance that helps to slow down digestion and keep you feeling fuller for longer. Sources of soluble fibre include oats, barley, fruits, vegetables, and legumes. Insoluble fibre does not dissolve in water, and instead passes through your digestive system largely unchanged. Sources of insoluble fibre include wheat bran, whole grains, and vegetables. Fibre is an important part of a healthy diet as it helps to keep your digestive system running smoothly. It helps to maintain regular bowel movements, prevents constipation, and can help lower cholesterol levels. Fibre can also help control blood sugar levels, reduce the risk of heart disease, and promote weight loss. Eating a diet that is high in fibre can help you get all of the benefits mentioned above. Aim to eat at least 25-30g of fibre per day. Try to include a variety of fibre-rich foods in your diet, such as fruits, vegetables, whole grains, nuts, and legumes. In addition to eating foods that are high in fibre, drinking plenty of water is also important. Water helps to keep your digestive system running smoothly and can help you to get the most out of the fibre in your diet. By eating a diet that is high in fibre and drinking plenty of water, you can help to keep your digestive system running smoothly and reap the many health benefits that fibre provides.

Fibre is an essential part of a healthy diet. It is a form of carbohydrate found in plant-based foods such as fruits, vegetables, grains, and legumes. Not all carbohydrates are created equal, however, and fibre is among the most beneficial for the body. Fibre has numerous health benefits, ranging from weight management to improved digestion, and is essential for maintaining a healthy gut. Fibre helps to regulate digestion and promote regularity. It helps to break down food, promoting regularity and reducing constipation. Fibre also helps to slow down digestion and can help to manage blood sugar levels, making it beneficial for those with diabetes. Fibre helps to keep the digestive system healthy and can help to reduce the risk of certain diseases, such as colon cancer. Fibre is also beneficial for weight management. It helps to keep you feeling full for longer, reducing the urge to snack or overeat. Fibre is also beneficial for weight management as it helps to regulate blood sugar levels, reducing the risk of developing type 2 diabetes. Fibre is also beneficial for heart health. It helps to reduce cholesterol levels and can help to reduce the risk of developing heart disease. Fibre helps to reduce inflammation, which can help to protect against certain types of cancer. Fibre is also beneficial for the immune system. It helps to provide essential vitamins and minerals to the body, which can help to boost the immune system and reduce the risk of infection. Fibre also helps to feed the beneficial bacteria in the gut, which can help to maintain a healthy balance of bacteria. Overall, fibre is an essential part of a healthy diet. It can help to regulate digestion, promote weight management, reduce cholesterol levels, boost the immune system, and reduce the risk of developing certain diseases. Eating a diet rich in fruits, vegetables, grains, and legumes is the best way to ensure you are getting enough fibre.

Best food sources

Fibre is an important part of a healthy diet. It helps keep your digestive system functioning properly, lowers cholesterol levels, and helps you feel full longer. It is found in plant-based foods and can be classified as either soluble or insoluble fibre. Soluble fibre absorbs water and slows digestion while insoluble fibre adds bulk to stools and helps them pass through the intestines more quickly. The best sources of fibre are.

Fruits

Fruits are one of the most important sources of dietary fibre. Fibre is an important part of a balanced diet, as it helps to promote regularity, lowers cholesterol, and helps maintain a healthy weight. While it may not be the most exciting part of a diet, it is essential for good health. Fruits are an excellent source of dietary fibre. Most fruits contain both soluble and insoluble fibre, though some may contain more of one than the other. Soluble fibre dissolves in water and helps to slow digestion, while insoluble fibre passes through the digestive tract relatively unchanged. Fruits are also high in vitamins and minerals, which makes them an important part of a healthy diet. For example, apples are a great source of fibre, as well as vitamin C, potassium, and magnesium. Berries, such as blueberries, contain high levels of fibre and antioxidants. In addition to providing fibre, fruits are also a great source of other essential nutrients such as vitamins, minerals, and antioxidants. For example, oranges are a great source of vitamin C, potassium, and folate. Bananas are rich in potassium, magnesium, and manganese. Fruits are also a great source of dietary fibre, which can help to lower cholesterol and promote regularity. Eating just one serving of fruit per day can provide up to 10% of the recommended daily fibre intake. Overall, fruits are an important part of a healthy diet. They are a great source of fibre, vitamins, minerals, and antioxidants. Eating a variety of fruits can help to ensure that you get all the essential nutrients your body needs.

Vegetables

Fibre is an essential component of a healthy diet and is found in a variety of plant-based foods, including vegetables. Vegetables are a great source of dietary fibre, which can help to regulate digestion, lower cholesterol levels, and reduce the risk of certain diseases. Fibre is a type of carbohydrate that cannot be broken down by the body, so it passes through the digestive system relatively unchanged. Vegetables are one of the best sources of dietary fibre. In fact, most non-starchy vegetables contain a significant amount of fibre. For example, one cup of broccoli contains 5 grams of fibre, one cup of cauliflower contains 2.5 grams of fibre, and one cup of Brussels sprouts contains 4 grams of fibre. Fibre is important for digestion because it helps to maintain a healthy balance of bacteria in the gut. Fibre helps to keep the digestive system running smoothly by adding bulk to stools and keeping them moving through the digestive tract. Fibre also helps to slow the absorption of sugar into the bloodstream, which can reduce spikes in blood sugar levels. Fibre has also been linked to a number of other health benefits. It can help to reduce cholesterol levels by binding to cholesterol-containing bile acids and carrying them out of the body. It can also help to reduce the risk of certain diseases, such as type 2 diabetes, heart disease, and certain types of cancer. In addition to providing fibre, vegetables are also rich in essential vitamins, minerals, and other nutrients. Eating a variety of vegetables can help to ensure that you get a wide range of these essential nutrients. To get the most out of your vegetables, it is important to prepare them in a way that preserves their nutritional value. Boiling and steaming are the best methods for cooking vegetables, as they retain the most nutrients. Avoid overcooking your vegetables, as this can reduce their nutritional value. In conclusion, vegetables are a great source of dietary fibre. Eating a variety of vegetables can provide you with the essential nutrients and fibre that your body needs for optimal health.

Nuts

Nuts are a great source of dietary fibre and are a popular snack for people of all ages. Dietary fibre is an important component of a healthy diet and is essential for proper digestion and overall health. Fibre is found in many foods, but nuts are particularly rich in it. Nuts are a good source of both soluble and insoluble fibre. Soluble fibre helps to reduce cholesterol levels, regulate blood sugar levels, and keep the digestive system healthy. Insoluble fibre helps to keep the intestines clean and reduce the risk of constipation. Both types of fibre are important for overall health. Nuts are high in fibre, with most containing between 2 and 7 grams per ounce. Almonds, cashews, and pistachios are among the highest in fibre content, with at least 2.5 grams per ounce. Walnuts, pecans, and macadamia nuts are slightly lower in fibre, with around 2 grams per ounce. Nuts are also a good source of other important nutrients such as protein, vitamin E, and healthy fats. Eating a handful of nuts as a snack is a great way to get the fibre and other nutrients you need. When snacking on nuts, it's important to keep in mind that they are high in calories and fat. Therefore, it's best to eat them in moderation. Eating too many nuts can lead to weight gain, so it's important to be mindful of portion sizes. Including nuts in your diet is an excellent way to get the fibre you need. Not only are they a great source of dietary fibre, but they are also a good source of other important nutrients. Eating a handful of nuts on a regular basis can help to keep your digestive system healthy, reduce cholesterol levels, and regulate blood sugar.

Seeds

One of the best sources of fibre is found in food seeds, such as flax and chia. Flax seeds are high in both soluble and insoluble fibre, making them beneficial for both digestion and heart health. They are also high in omega-3 fatty acids, which are important for brain health and overall well-being. Flax seeds can be eaten on their own, added to smoothies, or ground and added to breads and other baked goods. Chia seeds are also high in fibre, with about five grams of fibre per tablespoon. They are also high in protein and omega-3 fatty acids. Chia seeds can be eaten raw, added to smoothies or yogurt, or used in baking. Food seeds are also a great source of other nutrients, such as vitamins, minerals, and antioxidants. These nutrients can help reduce inflammation, boost the immune system, and protect against chronic diseases. Including food seeds in your diet is an easy and delicious way to get more fibre and other essential nutrients. They are also a great source of energy and can help keep you feeling full and satisfied. Try adding a tablespoon of flax or chia seeds to your morning smoothie or yogurt or sprinkling them over your favourite salad. You can also add them to baking recipes, such as muffins, breads, and cookies. Overall, food seeds are an excellent source of fibre, protein, and other essential nutrients. Eating them regularly can help promote regular digestion, improve heart health, and reduce your risk of certain diseases.

Whole Grains

Whole grains are an important part of a healthy diet, providing essential nutrients, fibre and a variety of other health benefits. Fibre is an important part of a healthy diet and can help promote good digestion and regularity. Whole grains are a great source of fibre, providing both soluble and insoluble types. Soluble fibre dissolves in water and is found in oats, barley, and some fruits, vegetables, and legumes. Soluble fibre helps to lower cholesterol, regulate blood sugar levels, and keep you feeling full for longer. It also helps to feed the beneficial bacteria in your gut, which helps with digestion and overall health. Insoluble fibre does not dissolve in water and is found in wheat, bran, nuts and some vegetables. Insoluble fibre helps to add bulk to your stool and keep you regular. It can also help to reduce your risk of developing certain types of cancer and reduce the risk of developing type 2 diabetes. Whole grains are a great source of both types of fibre. They are packed with nutrients, including B-vitamins, iron, magnesium, selenium and zinc. Whole grains are also low in fat, cholesterol and sodium, making them a great choice for a healthy diet. Whole grains can be incorporated into your diet in a variety of ways. You can add them to soups, salads and casseroles, use them to make your own bread and muffins, or even make hot cereal with them. Whole grains can also be used as a substitute for white rice or pasta in any dish. Eating a diet rich in whole grains and fibre is important for overall health and well-being. Whole grains are a great source of fibre and other essential nutrients and can help to keep you feeling full and regular. Incorporating whole grains into your diet can help to improve your health and may even reduce your risk of developing certain diseases.

VITAMINS

Vitamins are essential nutrients that the body needs to stay healthy and function properly. They are found in both animal and plant foods, as well as in dietary supplements. Vitamins are essential for a range of bodily functions, from forming new cells and enzymes, to maintaining bones, teeth, skin and hair. Vitamins can be divided into two categories: fat-soluble and water-soluble. Fat-soluble vitamins, such as vitamins A, D, E and K, are absorbed into the body's fat stores and can be used when needed. Water-soluble vitamins, such as vitamins B and C, are not stored in the body, so they must be consumed daily. Vitamin A is important for healthy vision, skin, and immune system. It is found in foods such as eggs, milk and cheese, as well as in dark, leafy green vegetables and orange, yellow, and red fruits and vegetables. Vitamin B complex is important for energy production, metabolism, and brain and nervous system function. It is found in foods such as whole grains, legumes, nuts and seeds, as well as in animal products such as eggs, milk and cheese. Vitamin C is important for healthy skin and bones, as well as for wound healing. It is found in citrus fruits, peppers, tomatoes, broccoli, and other fruits and vegetables. Vitamin D is important for strong bones and teeth, as well as for healthy skin, muscles, and nerves. It is found in foods such as fortified milk, eggs, and fatty fish. Vitamin E is important for healthy skin and eyes, as well as for maintaining healthy cells. It is found in foods such as nuts, seeds, and vegetable oils. Vitamin K is important for blood clotting, as well as for maintaining healthy bones. It is found in leafy green vegetables, as well as in some dairy products. Deficiencies in any of these vitamins can cause a range of health problems, from fatigue and muscle weakness to an increased risk of infection and even certain types of cancer. Therefore, it's important to make sure you're getting enough of the essential vitamins through the foods you eat, or by taking a multivitamin supplement.

Vitamins are essential for the body to function properly and maintain overall health. They're needed for a variety of body functions, including growth and development, the production of hormones, and the maintenance of strong bones and teeth. They're also important for the absorption of nutrients from food. Vitamins are divided into two groups: fat-soluble and water-soluble. Fat-soluble vitamins are stored in the body, while water-soluble vitamins need to be replenished regularly. Fat-soluble vitamins are important for a range of bodily functions. They help the body use proteins and carbohydrates, maintain healthy skin and vision, and build strong bones and teeth. Fat-soluble vitamins include vitamins A, D, E, and K. Water-soluble vitamins are important for a variety of metabolic processes. They help the body generate energy, maintain proper nerve and muscle function, and keep the immune system strong. Water-soluble vitamins include vitamins B and C. Vitamins are also important for maintaining a healthy weight. Many vitamins, such as vitamin B12, are essential for the body to break down and use the calories it takes in from food. Some vitamins, such as vitamin D, have been linked to increased weight loss. Vitamins can also help prevent certain health conditions, such as heart disease, stroke, and some forms of cancer. Vitamins B6, B12, and folate have been linked to a lower risk of cardiovascular disease, while vitamin C is thought to reduce the risk of certain types of cancer. Vitamins are an essential part of a healthy diet. They help the body function properly and maintain overall health. Eating a balanced diet that includes a variety of foods can help ensure you're getting all the vitamins and minerals you need. Taking a multivitamin supplement can also help fill in any nutritional gaps.

Vitamin A

Vitamin A is a fat-soluble vitamin found in many foods, including meat, poultry, fish, eggs, dairy products, and some plant-based foods, such as carrots and sweet potatoes. Vitamin A plays an important role in vision, bone growth, reproduction, and cell division. It is also a powerful antioxidant, which helps protect cells from damage caused by free radicals. Vitamin A is essential for healthy skin and eyes. It helps the eyes adjust to different levels of light and helps prevent night blindness. Vitamin A also helps maintain healthy teeth and bones, as well as the lining of the respiratory and digestive tracts. Foods that are rich in vitamin A include beef liver, salmon, tuna, eggs, milk, cheese, carrots, cantaloupe, spinach, and kale. Orange and yellow fruits and vegetables, and some vegetable oils also contain vitamin A. Vitamin A is important for overall health, so it is important to include a variety of foods in your diet that are rich in vitamin A. Eating a balanced diet that includes a variety of foods can help ensure that you are getting enough of this important vitamin.

Vitamin Bs

Vitamins B are a group of eight water soluble vitamins that are essential for a wide range of bodily functions. These vitamins are vital for proper metabolism, nervous system functioning and energy production. Each of the eight vitamins has a unique role, and all of them work together to ensure that the body is functioning at its best. The first of the eight vitamins is Vitamin B1, also known as Thiamine. This vitamin helps the body to break down carbohydrates and convert them into energy. It also helps to maintain healthy nerve cells and muscles. Vitamin B1 is found in a variety of foods, including whole grains, legumes, nuts, and seeds. The second vitamin is Vitamin B2, or Riboflavin. This vitamin helps to convert the food we eat into energy and helps to maintain healthy skin, eyes and hair. It can be found in milk, cheese, eggs, nuts, and green vegetables. Vitamin B3, or Niacin, is the third of the B vitamins. This vitamin helps to maintain healthy skin and nerves, and it also helps the body to break down fats and proteins. It can be found in chicken, fish, peanuts, mushrooms, and avocados. The fourth vitamin is Vitamin B5, or Pantothenic Acid. This vitamin helps to convert food into energy and helps to produce hormones. It can be found in meat, eggs, nuts, and legumes. The fifth vitamin is Vitamin B6, or Pyridoxine. This vitamin helps to keep the nervous system functioning properly and helps to produce red blood cells. It can be found in fish, bananas, potatoes, and some dark leafy green vegetables. The sixth vitamin is Vitamin B7, or Biotin. This vitamin helps to break down carbohydrates, fats and proteins, and it also helps to keep hair, skin and nails healthy. It can be found in eggs, salmon, nuts, and seeds. The seventh vitamin is Vitamin B9, or Folic Acid. This vitamin helps to produce red blood cells and helps to convert food into energy. It can be found in spinach, asparagus, beans, and some citrus fruits. The eighth vitamin is Vitamin B12, or Cobalamin. This vitamin helps to produce red blood cells and helps to maintain healthy nerve cells. It can be found in animal products, such as meat, fish, eggs, and milk.

Vitamin C

Vitamin C is an essential nutrient that the body needs to remain healthy. It is a water-soluble vitamin that is necessary for the production of collagen, which is a protein that helps in the formation of connective tissues, bones, cartilage, and skin. Vitamin C also plays a vital role in the absorption of minerals, including iron, and helps to boost the immune system. Vitamin C is found in a variety of fruits and vegetables and can also be taken in supplement form. Vitamin C is an antioxidant, meaning it helps to protect cells from damage caused by free radicals. Free radicals are atoms or molecules that can cause damage to our cells, leading to chronic diseases, such as cancer and heart disease. Vitamin C can help to neutralize free radicals and reduce their effects on our bodies. Vitamin C has a number of other health benefits as well. It helps to reduce inflammation, which can help with conditions such as arthritis and asthma. Vitamin C has also been found to reduce the risk of certain cancers, including lung cancer and stomach cancer. Vitamin C is also important for wound healing. It helps to stimulate the production of collagen, which is necessary for wound healing and tissue repair. Vitamin C also helps to reduce inflammation and swelling, which can help speed up the healing process. Vitamin C is found in a variety of foods, including citrus fruits, peppers, broccoli, strawberries, and leafy greens. It is also available in supplement form and can be taken as tablets or capsules. The recommended daily intake of vitamin C is 40-60mg per day. If you do not get enough vitamin C from your diet, you may need to take a supplement. It is important to talk to your doctor before taking any supplements to make sure they are safe for you. Overall, vitamin C is an essential nutrient that plays an important role in maintaining good health. Eating a variety of fruits and vegetables and taking supplements, if necessary, can help to ensure you get enough vitamin C every day.

Vitamin D

Vitamin D is an essential nutrient for overall health and well-being. It is a fat-soluble vitamin that helps the body absorb calcium, regulates the immune system, and helps maintain healthy bones, teeth, and skin. It is also important for regulating mood and energy levels. Vitamin D is produced naturally in our bodies when our skin is exposed to ultraviolet (UV) rays from the sun. Unfortunately, since many of us spend most of our time indoors, we don't get enough sunlight. This can lead to a vitamin D deficiency, which can cause a host of health problems. The recommended daily intake of vitamin D for adults is 600 IU (international units) per day. However, the amount of vitamin D you need can vary depending on your age, weight, and lifestyle. It's important to talk to your doctor to determine the right amount of vitamin D for you. Foods that are rich in vitamin D include fatty fish, such as salmon and tuna, as well as egg yolks, fortified milk, and fortified cereals. You can also get vitamin D through supplements, although it's important to talk to your doctor before taking any supplements. Vitamin D deficiency can lead to a variety of health problems, including weakened bones, an increased risk of infection, and depression. It can also lead to an increased risk of developing certain chronic illnesses, such as heart disease, diabetes, and cancer. If you think you may have a vitamin D deficiency, it's important to talk to your doctor. Your doctor can perform a blood test to determine your vitamin D levels and make recommendations for how to increase your intake of vitamin D. In summary, vitamin D is an essential nutrient for overall health and well-being. It is produced in our bodies when our skin is exposed to sunlight, but unfortunately, many of us don't get enough sunlight. Vitamins D supplements are available as well, but it is important to talk to your doctor before taking any supplements. A vitamin D deficiency can lead to a variety of health problems, so if you think you may have a vitamin D deficiency, it's important to talk to your doctor.

Vitamin E

Vitamin E is a fat-soluble vitamin that is essential for human health. It is a powerful antioxidant that helps protect cells from damage caused by free radicals. Vitamin E also plays a role in maintaining healthy skin, eyes, and immune system. Vitamin E is found in a variety of foods, including nuts, seeds, vegetable oils, leafy greens, and fortified cereals. It is also available in dietary supplement form. Vitamin E plays an important role in protecting the body from oxidative damage. Oxidative damage occurs when free radicals, which are molecules with an unpaired electron, interact with cells. Free radicals damage cells and can lead to diseases such as cancer and heart disease. Vitamin

E helps protect cells from oxidative damage by neutralizing free radicals. Vitamin E is also necessary for maintaining healthy skin. It helps protect skin cells from damage caused by ultraviolet (UV) radiation. Vitamin E also helps reduce inflammation, which can help reduce the appearance of wrinkles and other signs of aging. Vitamin E is also important for eye health. It helps protect the eyes from damage caused by blue light, which can lead to age-related macular degeneration. Vitamin E also helps reduce the risk of cataracts. Vitamin E is also necessary for maintaining a healthy immune system. It helps regulate the body's inflammatory response and helps protect cells from oxidative damage. Vitamin E also helps boost the activity of certain immune cells, which can help the body fight off infections. In general, a healthy diet should provide enough vitamin E to meet your body's needs. If you don't get enough vitamin E in your diet, a supplement may be beneficial. Vitamin E supplements are available in both natural and synthetic forms. It is important to talk to your doctor before taking any supplements to make sure they are safe for you.

Vitamin Ks

Vitamin K is an essential nutrient required for proper blood clotting, bone and cardiovascular health. It is a fat-soluble vitamin, which means that it is stored in the body's fatty tissue, and it can be found in a variety of foods. Vitamin K helps to regulate the body's calcium levels, which is important for bone health, and it also helps to protect against excessive bleeding and other cardiovascular problems. The two major forms of vitamin K are vitamin K1, also known as phylloquinone, and vitamin K2, also known as menaquinone. Vitamin K1 is found naturally in green leafy vegetables, such as kale, spinach, and broccoli, as well as in vegetable oils and some fruits. Vitamin K2 is synthesized by bacteria in the human intestine, and is also found in fermented foods like cheese, yogurt, and natto. Vitamin K plays an important role in the body's clotting process. It helps to activate the proteins involved in blood clotting, which helps to stop bleeding when the body is injured. Without enough vitamin K, the body is unable to form clots, which can lead to excessive bleeding. Vitamin K also helps to regulate calcium levels in the body, which is important for maintaining strong bones and teeth. In addition, vitamin K has been linked to a number of other health benefits. Some studies suggest that it may help to reduce the risk of certain types of cancer, as well as reduce the risk of heart disease and stroke. It may also help to reduce the risk of osteoporosis and improve bone health. Most people get enough vitamin K through their diet, but some people may need to take vitamin K supplements to ensure they are getting enough. If you are pregnant or breastfeeding, you should talk to your doctor before taking any supplements. In general, it is recommended that adults get 90 micrograms of vitamin K each day. The best way to get enough vitamin K is to eat a variety of foods that are rich in the vitamin, such as green leafy vegetables, vegetable oils, and some fruits. If you are concerned about your vitamin K levels, talk to your doctor about taking supplements.

HERBS AND SPICES

Herbs and spices are the fragrant and flavourful ingredients that can turn a simple dish into a delicious culinary experience. Herbs and spices have been used for centuries to add flavour to food, enhance its nutrition, and even to treat medical conditions. Herbs are the leaves of an edible plant, either fresh or dried. Common herbs include basil, oregano, parsley, thyme, rosemary, and dill. These herbs are used to flavour a wide range of dishes from soups, sauces, and dressings to pasta, rice, and vegetables. Spices, on the other hand, are made from the seeds, bark, roots, and fruits of certain plants. Common spices include cinnamon, nutmeg, pepper, ginger, and cumin. Spices are used to add an extra layer of flavour to dishes such as curries, stews, and marinades. Herbs and spices are packed with antioxidants, vitamins, and minerals. They can help to reduce inflammation, boost the immune system, and even help with digestion. They may also help to reduce the risk of certain diseases and improve overall health. Herbs and spices can also be used to replace salt, which is high in sodium and can increase the risk of high blood pressure. By using herbs and spices, you can reduce your sodium intake and enjoy flavourful dishes without the added salt. When using herbs and spices, it is important to store them properly. Herbs and spices should be stored in an airtight container away from heat, sunlight, and moisture. They should also be kept away from strong-smelling foods such as onion and garlic, as the smell can be transferred to the herbs and spices. When cooking with herbs and spices, it is important to remember that a little goes a long way. Start with a small amount and add more to taste. Herbs and spices can also be combined in order to create unique flavours. Herbs and spices are a great way to add flavour and nutrition to any dish. With just a few simple ingredients, you can turn an ordinary meal into something special.

Herbs and spices are some of the healthiest foods on the planet. They are packed with antioxidants, minerals, vitamins, and other essential nutrients that can help protect your body from a variety of diseases and ailments. They can also be used to add flavour and nutrition to any meal. Here are some of the reasons why herbs and spices are good for the body. First, herbs and spices are high in antioxidants. Antioxidants are molecules that can help protect the body from harmful free radical molecules that can cause damage to cells and DNA. By consuming herbs and spices, you can help fight this damage, reduce inflammation, and promote healthy aging. Second, herbs and spices are rich in vitamins and minerals. Many herbs and spices are excellent sources of vitamins A, C, and E, as well as essential minerals such as zinc, iron, and magnesium. These vitamins and minerals can bolster your immune system, help maintain healthy bones, and assist in wound healing. Third, herbs and spices can help improve digestion. Many herbs and spices, such as ginger, turmeric, and cumin, can help improve digestive health by reducing inflammation and stimulating digestion. This can help prevent digestive issues like bloating, cramping, and constipation. Fourth, herbs and spices can help improve cognitive function. Many herbs and spices, such as rosemary and sage, are high in compounds like rosmarinic acid and thymol, which have been found to improve memory and concentration. Finally, herbs and spices can help reduce your risk of chronic disease. Studies have shown that regular consumption of herbs and spices can help reduce your risk of heart disease, cancer, and other chronic diseases. Herbs and spices are some of the healthiest foods you can consume. They are packed with essential vitamins and minerals, can help improve digestion and cognitive function, and can even reduce your risk of chronic disease. By incorporating more herbs and spices into your meals, you can reap the many benefits they have to offer.

Herbs and spices are an essential part of any kitchen. They add flavour and depth to many dishes, allowing cooks to create a variety of delectable meals. With such a wide range of herbs and spices available, it can be difficult to keep track of them all. Fortunately, there are hundreds of different herbs and spices to choose from – each with their own distinct flavour and aroma. Herbs are typically used in their fresh form, although dried versions are also available. Common herbs include basil, oregano, thyme, and bay leaves. Herbs are often used in Mediterranean cuisine, as well as in soups and sauces. Spices, on the other hand, are usually used in dried form, although some can be purchased fresh. Common spices include pepper, cinnamon, nutmeg, and cloves. Spices can be used to add flavour to a variety of dishes, from curries to desserts. In total, there are approximately 500 different herbs and spices available. Popular herbs and spices include.

Black Pepper

Black pepper is a spice commonly found in kitchens around the world. It is one of the most widely used spices for cooking and is an essential ingredient in many dishes. But did you know that black pepper is more than just a tasty addition to your meals? This humble spice is packed with health benefits that can improve your overall wellbeing. Black pepper contains a compound called piperine, which is responsible for its strong flavour. This compound is also known for its anti-inflammatory properties and its ability to boost the absorption of other nutrients. It can improve digestion, reduce cholesterol levels, and increase the body's metabolism. In addition to its effects on digestion, black pepper also has antioxidant properties. This means that it can help protect the body's cells from damage caused by free radicals. This could help reduce the risk of chronic diseases like cancer and heart disease. Black pepper can also help relieve pain and discomfort. It contains a compound called capsaicin, which is the same compound that gives chili peppers their heat. When applied topically, capsaicin can reduce pain and inflammation. Finally, black pepper can help boost the immune system. It contains vitamin C, which can help fight off infections and boost the body's defences. It also contains zinc, which is necessary for the proper functioning of the immune system. Overall, black pepper is a powerful spice with numerous health benefits. It can improve digestion, reduce inflammation, and boost the immune system. So, why not add some to your meals and reap the benefits?

Cinnamon

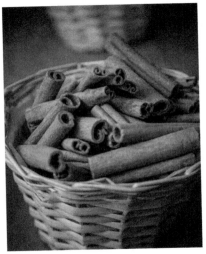

Cinnamon is a well-known spice, commonly used in baking, that is derived from the inner bark of several different trees. It has a sweet and spicy flavour that can be used to enhance both sweet and savoury dishes. Cinnamon has been used as a medicinal herb for centuries and has a long list of potential health benefits. Cinnamon is a great source of antioxidants, which helps protect the body from oxidative stress and free radical damage. Studies have shown that cinnamon can help reduce inflammation and oxidative damage caused by diabetes, as well as reduce blood sugar levels. It has also been linked to improving cholesterol levels and reducing the risk of heart disease. Cinnamon is also thought to have antibacterial and antifungal properties, which can help protect against infections and fight against bacteria and fungi. It has also been found to be beneficial in treating nausea, indigestion, and stomach ache. Cinnamon has also been shown to help reduce menstrual cramps and may also help reduce the risk of certain cancers. Cinnamon is also thought to have anti-inflammatory properties, which can help reduce the risk of arthritis, asthma, and other inflammatory conditions. It can also help reduce the symptoms of colds and flu and may even help reduce the severity of allergies. Cinnamon is also a great source of vitamins and minerals, including calcium, iron, magnesium, and zinc. It is also a good source of dietary fibre, which can help improve digestion and provide energy to the body. Overall, cinnamon is a great addition to any diet. It is a delicious, low-calorie spice that can provide a wide range of health benefits. It can help reduce inflammation, improve cholesterol levels, reduce the risk of certain cancers, reduce the severity of colds and flu, and provide the body with essential vitamins and minerals. Make sure to include cinnamon in your diet today to enjoy all of its amazing health benefits.

Sage

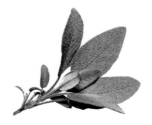

Sage is a popular herb that has been used in traditional medicine for centuries. It is a member of the mint family and has a strong, aromatic flavour. Sage is used in a variety of culinary dishes and is also known for its medicinal properties. Sage is packed with nutrients and antioxidants that can help promote good health. It contains vitamins A and K, as well as minerals like calcium, magnesium, and zinc. It also contains polyphenols, which are compounds that can protect against free radical damage and reduce inflammation. Sage is known for its ability to improve cognitive function. It has been used as a natural remedy for Alzheimer's disease and dementia, as well as memory loss. Studies have shown that consuming sage can improve memory and concentration. Sage can also be beneficial for digestive health. It has been used to treat indigestion, nausea, and excessive gas. Sage can also help reduce the symptoms of irritable bowel syndrome (IBS). Sage is known for its anti-inflammatory properties. It has been used to treat a variety of conditions associated with inflammation, including arthritis, asthma, and eczema. Sage has also been used to reduce the symptoms of colds, flu, and sore throats. Sage can also help improve mood and reduce stress. It contains compounds that may help reduce anxiety and depression. Studies have shown that it can improve mood and reduce symptoms of stress. Sage is also beneficial for skin health. It can help reduce acne and wrinkles, as well as improve overall skin tone. It can also help reduce redness and swelling. Overall, sage is a powerful herb that can provide numerous health benefits. It can help improve cognitive function, digestive health, and mood. It can also help reduce inflammation and improve skin health. For these reasons, sage is a great addition to any diet.

Turmeric

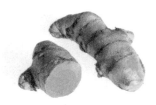

Turmeric is a popular spice that is derived from the turmeric plant and has been used in traditional Indian and Chinese medicine for centuries. It's also used in many culinary dishes due to its vibrant orange-yellow colour and earthy flavour.

However, Turmeric is much more than just a flavourful spice, as it has numerous health benefits. Turmeric contains a compound called curcumin, which is the active ingredient in the spice and is responsible for many of its health benefits. Curcumin is a powerful anti-inflammatory and antioxidant, which can help to reduce inflammation in the body, reduce oxidative damage and improve overall health. It can also help reduce the risk of certain diseases, such as heart disease, cancer and Alzheimer's disease. Studies have found that curcumin can help to reduce cholesterol, improve blood sugar levels, and reduce symptoms of depression and anxiety. Turmeric can also help to boost the immune system, as it has anti-bacterial and anti-viral properties. It can help to fight off infections and reduce the risk of getting sick. Turmeric can also help to improve digestion and reduce digestive issues, such as bloating and gas. It can also help to reduce the risk of certain digestive diseases, such as ulcerative colitis and Crohn's disease. In addition, turmeric can help to improve skin health, as it can reduce inflammation and help to prevent wrinkles and age spots. Overall, turmeric is a powerful spice that has numerous health benefits. It can help to reduce inflammation, boost the immune system, reduce the risk of certain diseases, improve digestion and skin health. Therefore, adding turmeric to your diet can help to improve your overall health and well-being.

Basil

Basil is an herb that has been used for centuries as both a culinary and medicinal plant. It has long been valued for its healing properties and is considered to be a natural remedy for a variety of ailments. It is thought to be beneficial for the body, mind and spirit. Basil is rich in vitamins, minerals, and antioxidants, which makes it an ideal choice for those looking to boost their overall health. It contains vitamins A, C and K, as well as manganese, magnesium, iron and calcium. It has also been found to contain a number of essential oils, including eugenol and estragole, which are believed to have anti-inflammatory and antimicrobial properties. Basil is known to have a positive effect on the digestive system. It can help to boost the metabolism and aid in digestion, as well as relieve constipation, bloating and gas. It is also believed to help reduce nausea and vomiting and is often used to treat stomach aches, cramps and indigestion. Basil has been found to have antioxidant and anti-inflammatory properties, which can help to reduce inflammation and protect against oxidative damage. It is thought to be beneficial for the respiratory system, helping to reduce symptoms of asthma and bronchitis. It can also help to reduce allergies and boost the immune system. Basil is believed to have a calming and soothing effect on the body and is often used to help relieve stress and anxiety. It can help to improve sleep and provide a sense of mental clarity and well-being. Basil can also be used to help improve the health of the skin. It is thought to help reduce the appearance of wrinkles and fine lines, as well as help heal wounds and burns. It is also believed to have antiseptic properties, which can help to prevent infection and reduce the risk of skin infections. Overall, basil is a powerful herb that has been used for centuries for its healing properties. It is rich in vitamins, minerals, and antioxidants and is believed to help improve digestion, reduce inflammation, boost the immune system, reduce stress and anxiety, and improve the health of the skin.

Parsley

Parsley is a popular herb that is widely used in many dishes around the world. It is known for its distinctive flavour and bright green colour. It is also packed with many health benefits that can help improve your overall health. Parsley is rich in vitamins and minerals, such as vitamins A, C, K, and E. It also contains a variety of other nutrients, including folate, iron, magnesium, and potassium. All of these vitamins and minerals play a role in keeping your body healthy and functioning properly. Parsley is a great source of antioxidants, which can help protect your cells from damage caused by free radicals. Free radicals are molecules that can cause damage to cells, which can lead to disease. Antioxidants help neutralize these molecules and protect your cells. Parsley is also high in fibre, which can help keep your digestive system running smoothly. Fibre helps add bulk to your stools and makes them easier to pass. Additionally, fibre helps keep your blood sugar levels stable, which can help prevent diabetes. Parsley is also a good source of folic acid, which is important for pregnant women. Folic acid helps prevent birth defects, such as spina bifida. It also helps form red blood cells and helps the body use protein and fat. Parsley also has anti-inflammatory properties. Inflammation is the body's natural response to injury or infection, but it can also contribute to the development of chronic diseases. Parsley can help reduce inflammation and may help relieve symptoms of arthritis and other inflammatory conditions. Parsley is also rich in polyphenols, which are plant compounds that have powerful anti-cancer properties. Polyphenols have been shown to reduce the risk of certain types of cancer, including colon, stomach, and breast cancer. In conclusion, parsley is a popular herb that is packed with many health benefits. It is rich in vitamins, minerals, and antioxidants, which can help protect your cells from damage and help keep your digestive system running smoothly. Additionally, parsley is a good source of folic acid, which is important for pregnant women, and it also has anti-inflammatory and anti-cancer properties. For these reasons, it is a great addition to any diet.

Cayenne Pepper

Cayenne pepper is a popular spice with a variety of culinary and medicinal uses. Its spicy flavour comes from a compound called capsaicin, which is believed to have many health benefits. In this article, we'll explore the potential health benefits of cayenne pepper. Cayenne pepper has been used in traditional medicine for centuries. It's thought to have anti-inflammatory, antioxidant, and pain-relieving properties. In addition, some research suggests that it may help with weight loss, digestive health, and heart health. Cayenne pepper is rich in capsaicin, a compound that gives it its spicy flavour. Capsaicin is thought to reduce inflammation and provide pain relief. It's also believed to be an antioxidant, which means it may help protect cells from damage caused by free radicals. Cayenne pepper may also help with weight loss. A study in rats found that capsaicin helped reduce food intake and body weight. It may also speed up metabolism, which can help you burn more calories. Cayenne pepper is also thought to improve digestion. It may help stimulate digestive enzymes and increase the secretion of stomach acid. This may help break down food more efficiently and improve nutrient absorption. Cayenne pepper may also help improve heart health. A study in rats found that capsaicin reduced total cholesterol, LDL cholesterol, and triglycerides. It also increased levels of HDL, or "good" cholesterol. Overall, cayenne pepper is a popular spice with a variety of potential health benefits. It may help reduce inflammation, aid in weight loss, improve digestion, and support heart health. More research is needed to confirm these effects in humans.

Ginger

Ginger is one of the most widely used and versatile spices in the world. It has been used for thousands of years in many cultures for both culinary and medicinal purposes. This powerful root is chock-full of health benefits, ranging from helping to reduce inflammation to aiding digestion. Here are just some of the wonderful health benefits of ginger:

1. Anti-inflammatory: Ginger has powerful anti-inflammatory properties, which can help reduce pain and swelling associated with conditions like arthritis and muscle soreness. It can also help reduce inflammation in the gut and has been used to treat inflammatory bowel diseases like Crohn's and ulcerative colitis.

2. Digestion: Ginger has been used for centuries to aid digestion and to treat digestive issues like nausea, vomiting, and upset stomach. It can help reduce bloating and gas and can even help

stimulate the production of bile, which helps break down fats.

3. Heart Health: Ginger is rich in antioxidants, which can help protect against heart disease, stroke, and other cardiovascular problems. It can also reduce cholesterol levels and help lower blood pressure.

4. Immunity: Ginger has been used for centuries to help boost the immune system and to fight off colds and flu. It can also help reduce the severity of symptoms associated with respiratory illnesses.

5. Pain Relief: Ginger has been used for centuries to help reduce pain and inflammation, particularly in the joints. It can help reduce muscle and joint pain associated with arthritis and can even help reduce the severity of headache pain.

Ginger is an incredibly powerful and versatile spice with a wide range of health benefits. Whether you're looking for relief from digestive issues, inflammation, or pain, it's a great natural remedy to try.

Garlic

Garlic is one of the world's most popular ingredients, used in cooking around the world. It adds flavour to food, but it is also packed with health benefits. Studies have shown that garlic can help reduce the risk of many diseases and ailments, from heart disease to cancer. Here are some of the health benefits of garlic.

1. It lowers cholesterol: Studies have shown that garlic can help lower cholesterol levels by reducing the amount of bad cholesterol (LDL) in the body. It also increases the amount of good cholesterol (HDL).

2. It helps reduce blood pressure: Garlic can help reduce blood pressure by relaxing the blood vessels, which allows for better blood flow.

3. It boosts the immune system: Garlic contains compounds that can help boost the immune system and fight off viruses and bacteria.

4. It helps fight off colds and flu: Garlic has antiviral properties that can help fight off colds and flu. It can also reduce the severity of symptoms.

5. It helps reduce inflammation: Garlic contains compounds that can help reduce inflammation in the body. This can help reduce the risk of many diseases, such as arthritis and Alzheimer's.

6. It helps protect against cancer: Garlic contains compounds that can help protect against certain types of cancer, including stomach, colon, and prostate cancer.

7. It has anti-aging benefits: Garlic contains antioxidants that can help protect the body from the effects of aging.

Garlic is a powerful ingredient that can have a positive effect on your health. It can help reduce cholesterol and blood pressure, boost the immune system, fight off colds and flu, reduce inflammation, and even protect against cancer. Adding garlic to your diet can help you enjoy all of these health benefits.

Peppermint

Peppermint is a popular flavour of tea, gum, and candy, but it also has a number of health benefits that make it a valuable addition to your diet. Peppermint oil, which is derived from the leaves of the peppermint plant, is known for its medicinal properties. The most well-known benefit of peppermint is its ability to soothe digestive issues, such as indigestion, constipation, and nausea. Peppermint oil can be taken in capsule form or added to tea to help reduce symptoms. Research has shown that peppermint oil can relax the muscles of the digestive tract, allowing for easier passage of food and waste. This can help to alleviate the symptoms associated with irritable bowel syndrome (IBS). Peppermint oil has also been found to be an effective treatment for headaches and migraines. Studies have shown that peppermint oil applied topically to the temples and forehead can reduce the intensity of headache pain. Peppermint oil can also be inhaled or taken in capsule form to help reduce the frequency and duration of migraine attacks. Peppermint is a type of mint plant that has been used for centuries for its medicinal properties, making it a popular choice for home remedies. It is known for its refreshing and calming aroma, and for the health benefits it may provide. The most beneficial compounds in peppermint are menthol, menthone, and menthyl acetate. These compounds are known to have anti-inflammatory and antimicrobial properties, which can help to soothe a sore throat, reduce congestion, and ease other symptoms of colds and flu. Menthol can also reduce muscle tension and relieve pain associated with headaches, migraines, and arthritis. In addition to its anti-inflammatory properties, peppermint has been found to improve digestive health. Its menthol content can relax the muscles in the digestive tract, which can help to reduce bloating, nausea, and other gastrointestinal issues. It can also help to reduce the symptoms of irritable bowel syndrome, such as abdominal pain and cramping. The menthol in peppermint may also have a calming effect on the mind. Studies have shown that the scent of peppermint can help to boost energy levels and improve concentration. It can also help to reduce stress and promote relaxation. its digestive and headache-relieving properties, peppermint oil has also been found to have antimicrobial and anti-inflammatory properties. This means it can help to fight off bacteria and viruses and reduce inflammation in the body. It can help to reduce the symptoms of asthma, as well as reduce acne and other skin conditions. Peppermint offers a variety of health benefits and is an easy addition to any diet. Whether you choose to drink peppermint tea, add peppermint oil to your skincare routine, or simply enjoy the scent of this popular herb, you can reap the rewards of its medicinal properties.

Rosemary

Rosemary is an herb that is native to the Mediterranean region. It has a distinctive, pungent smell and flavour and is commonly used in cooking. But did you know that rosemary has some incredible health benefits as well? Here are just a few of them:

1. Improved Brain Function: Rosemary has been studied for its ability to improve cognitive function. Studies have found that ingesting rosemary can improve memory, concentration, and focus. It also may help reduce stress and anxiety.

2. Improved Digestion: Rosemary has been used to treat digestive problems for centuries. It can help to stimulate the production of bile, which helps to break down fats and other nutrients in the digestive tract. It can also act as a natural laxative, helping to move waste through the digestive system.

3. Improved Immunity: Rosemary is rich in antioxidants, which help to protect the body from free radicals that can cause damage to cells. Rosemary also contains anti-inflammatory compounds that can help reduce inflammation in the body.

4. Improved Bone Health: Rosemary is a great source of Vitamin A, which helps to strengthen bones and prevent bone loss. It also contains calcium, magnesium, and phosphorus, which are all important for healthy bones.

5. Improved Skin Health: Rosemary has been found to have anti-aging properties. It can help to reduce wrinkles and fine lines and can help to protect the skin from damage. It also contains Vitamin E, which can help to keep the skin hydrated and supple. These are just a few of the health benefits of rosemary. Whether you're using it to add flavour to a dish or to reap the health benefits, it's a great addition to your diet.

Fenugreek

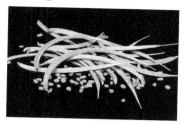

Fenugreek is a plant that has been used for centuries to treat a variety of health issues, from digestive troubles to skin conditions. In recent years, studies have found that fenugreek can offer a variety of health benefits. Fenugreek is a rich source of vitamins and minerals, including Vitamin B6, Vitamin K, and potassium. It is also a good source of fibre, which can help to regulate digestion and keep the digestive system running smoothly. Eating fenugreek can also help to lower cholesterol levels and reduce the risk of heart disease. Additionally, fenugreek contains powerful antioxidants, which can help to protect the body from free radicals and reduce inflammation. Fenugreek has also been found to be beneficial for people with diabetes. The plant is thought to be able to reduce blood sugar levels and improve the body's sensitivity to insulin, helping to regulate blood glucose levels. Fenugreek may also help to reduce the risk of complications associated with diabetes, such as nerve damage and kidney disease. Fenugreek is also thought to have numerous benefits for women's health. It has been used as an herbal remedy to help with menstrual cramps and other menstrual-related conditions. Fenugreek is an ancient spice that has been used for centuries in Ayurvedic and Chinese medicine. It is a powerful medicinal herb that has been used to treat a variety of ailments, including digestive disorders, respiratory problems, skin conditions, and even diabetes. In recent years, research has also revealed that fenugreek has numerous health benefits and can be used to promote overall health and well-being. One of the most notable health benefits of fenugreek is its ability to improve digestion and reduce gastrointestinal discomfort. The herb is rich in dietary fibre and mucilage, both of which can help to reduce inflammation, improve digestion, and reduce constipation. Additionally, fenugreek contains compounds that can help to reduce the symptoms of irritable bowel syndrome (IBS) and other digestive disorders. Fenugreek is also believed to have anti-inflammatory properties, which can be beneficial for people suffering from arthritis and other inflammatory conditions. The compounds in fenugreek are thought to reduce the body's production of inflammatory compounds, which can help to reduce pain and swelling. Fenugreek is also high in antioxidants, which can help to protect the body from the damage caused by free radicals. It is also believed to have anti-cancer properties and may even be able to reduce the risk of certain types of cancer. Additionally, it is high in vitamins A, C, and K, which can help to improve the immune system.

AYURVEDIC HERBS AND SPICES

Ayurvedic herbs and spices are a type of natural medicine that has been used for centuries in India. They are made up of a variety of herbs and spices and are designed to help balance the body's energies and promote health and wellbeing. Ayurvedic herbs and spices are believed to have a variety of healing properties. They are used to treat a range of conditions, from digestive issues to skin conditions, to mental health issues. They can also be used to boost energy, support the immune system, and improve overall health. Ayurvedic herbs and spices are typically used as part of a holistic approach to health and wellbeing. They are often combined with other natural remedies, such as massage, yoga, and meditation, to increase their effectiveness. Common ayurvedic herbs and spices include turmeric, ginger, black pepper, cardamom, fennel, coriander, cinnamon, and cumin. Each of these herbs and spices has its own unique properties, and they are usually combined to create a powerful combination of healing properties. Turmeric is a common ayurvedic herb, and is known for its anti-inflammatory, antioxidant, and anti-bacterial properties. It is used to treat a variety of conditions, including indigestion, skin conditions, and joint pain. Ginger is another important ayurvedic herb and is known for its anti-nausea and anti-inflammatory properties. It can be used to improve digestion and reduce inflammation. Black pepper is a powerful ayurvedic spice, and is known for its anti-inflammatory, antioxidant, and antiseptic properties. It can help to reduce pain, improve circulation, and fight infection. Cardamom is a fragrant ayurvedic spice and is known for its digestive and calming properties. It is often used to treat indigestion, nausea, and stomach cramps. Fennel is an aromatic ayurvedic herb and is known for its anti-inflammatory and antioxidant properties. It can be used to treat a variety of conditions, including indigestion and respiratory issues. Coriander is a versatile ayurvedic herb and is known for its anti-inflammatory and digestive properties. It can be used to treat a variety of conditions, including indigestion and skin conditions. Cinnamon is a warming ayurvedic spice and is known for its anti-inflammatory and antioxidant properties. It can be used to treat a variety of conditions, including digestive issues, skin conditions, and joint pain. Cumin is a pungent ayurvedic spice and is known for its digestive and anti-inflammatory properties. It can be used to treat a variety of conditions, including indigestion and respiratory issues. Ayurvedic herbs and spices can be taken in a variety of forms, including teas, tinctures, and capsules. It is important to talk to a healthcare professional before taking any herbs or spices, as they can interact with medications and cause side effects.

Ayurvedic herbs and spices have been used for centuries to promote holistic health. In Ayurveda, the ancient Indian science of life, herbs and spices are used to balance the three doshas in the body - Vata, Pitta and Kapha. These three doshas represent the energy in the body and when they are in balance, it leads to good health. Ayurvedic herbs and spices are known to be very beneficial for overall health. They contain active compounds that act as powerful healing agents. They are often used to treat and prevent a variety of illnesses and conditions, ranging from digestive issues to skin issues. Many of these herbs and spices have anti-inflammatory and antioxidant properties, which can help to reduce inflammation in the body, reduce oxidative stress, and protect against disease. They can also help to boost the immune system, reduce fatigue, and improve the body's overall health. Ayurvedic herbs and spices are also known to help balance hormones and improve digestion. They can help to reduce bloating, constipation, and other digestive issues. They can also help to improve the absorption of nutrients from food, which can lead to better overall health. Many of these herbs and spices have also been shown to have anti-carcinogenic properties. They can help protect against cancer-causing agents and reduce the risk of developing certain types of cancer. Finally, these herbs and spices can be used to promote overall wellbeing. They can help to reduce stress, improve sleep, and promote relaxation. They can also help to regulate mood, reduce anxiety, and improve mental clarity. Overall, Ayurvedic herbs and spices are a great way to promote holistic health. They can help to balance the body's energy, reduce inflammation, and protect against disease. They can also help to improve digestion, boost the immune system, and promote overall wellbeing.

Ashwagandha

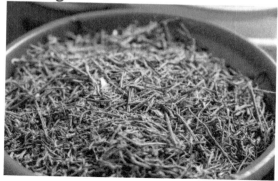

Ashwagandha is an ancient herb that has been used for thousands of years in Ayurvedic medicine. It is considered one of the most important herbs in Ayurveda and is known for its healing and energizing properties. Its scientific name is Withania somnifera, and it is also known as Indian Ginseng. Ashwagandha is an adaptogen, which means it helps the body adapt to stress. It can help boost energy levels, reduce fatigue, and improve concentration. It's also known for its anti-inflammatory and antioxidant properties, which can help protect against certain diseases. One of the most significant benefits of Ashwagandha is its ability to reduce stress and anxiety. Studies have shown that it can reduce cortisol levels and improve mood. It has also been found to reduce symptoms of depression and improve sleep quality. Ashwagandha can also help improve cognitive function by increasing memory and concentration. It can also help reduce symptoms of Alzheimer's and Parkinson's diseases. In addition to its mental health benefits, Ashwagandha can also help improve physical health. It can help reduce inflammation and boost the immune system. It can also help reduce cholesterol levels and improve cardiovascular health. Lastly, Ashwagandha can help reduce the side effects of chemotherapy and radiation. It can help improve overall quality of life in cancer patients. Overall, Ashwagandha is an incredibly powerful and beneficial herb that can help improve both mental and physical health. It can help reduce stress and anxiety, improve cognitive function, reduce inflammation, and boost the immune system. It can also help reduce the side effects of chemotherapy and radiation. For these reasons, it is an important herb for anyone looking to improve their overall health and wellbeing.

Cardamom

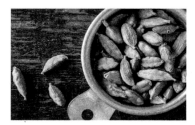

Cardamom is an aromatic spice with a unique flavour and a variety of health benefits. The small, round pods contain fragrant seeds that are used to flavour many dishes and drinks around the world. In addition to its culinary uses, cardamom is also known for its medicinal properties. Here are some of the health benefits of cardamom: Cardamom helps improve digestion by stimulating the secretion of digestive juices and relieving indigestion, bloating, and gas. It also helps to reduce acidity and heartburn. Cardamom can also be beneficial in treating irritable bowel syndrome and other digestive problems. Cardamom can help to boost the immune system by increasing the body's ability to fight off infections. It is known to have anti-inflammatory, anti-viral and anti-bacterial properties that can help protect the body from various illnesses. Cardamom can help to lower blood pressure and cholesterol levels. It is believed to reduce the risk of cardiovascular diseases by promoting healthy circulation and protecting the heart. It can also help to reduce the risk of stroke and other cardiovascular problems. Cardamom has been used for centuries to treat respiratory problems. It is known to be effective in relieving symptoms of asthma, bronchitis, and other respiratory disorders. Cardamom can also help to reduce congestion and soothe sore throats. Cardamom can help to improve oral health by reducing bad breath and promoting healthy teeth and gums. It is also known to have antiseptic properties that can help to prevent tooth decay and other oral infections. Cardamom is known to be a natural breath freshener and can help to reduce bad breath. It is also believed to have detoxifying properties that can help to remove toxins from the body and improve overall health. Cardamom can also be beneficial for skin health. It is known to have antioxidant properties that can help to reduce wrinkles and protect the skin from damage. It can also help to improve skin tone and complexion. These are just a few of the many health benefits of cardamom. This fragrant spice can be used to add flavour to food, but it can also be used for its medicinal properties. Cardamom can be taken in a variety of forms, including capsules, teas, and essential oils. If you are looking for a natural way to improve your health, cardamom is definitely worth a try.

Curcumin

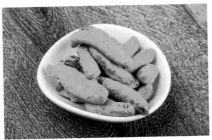

Curcumin is a powerful antioxidant found in the spice turmeric. It has been used in traditional medicine for centuries, and modern studies have revealed a variety of health benefits that it can offer. Curcumin has anti-inflammatory properties, which can help reduce inflammation associated with arthritis and other forms of joint pain. This can help reduce pain and improve mobility. Curcumin has also been shown to reduce the risk of heart disease by lowering cholesterol levels and reducing blood pressure. Curcumin has powerful antioxidant properties, which can help protect cells from damage. This can reduce the risk of certain types of cancer and can also help slow down the aging process. In addition, curcumin can help protect the liver from toxins, and can even help reduce the risk of Alzheimer's disease. Curcumin can also help improve digestion and reduce bloating and gas. It can help reduce nausea and vomiting and can even help reduce the symptoms of irritable bowel syndrome. Finally, curcumin can help boost the immune system, which can help protect the body from infection and disease. It can also help reduce stress and improve mood. Overall, curcumin is a powerful antioxidant with a variety of health benefits. It can help reduce inflammation, protect cells from damage, improve digestion, boost the immune system, and reduce stress and anxiety. For these reasons, it is an excellent addition to any diet, and can help improve overall health and wellbeing.

Boswellia

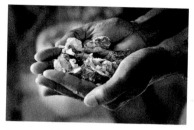

Boswellia, also known as Indian frankincense, is a tree native to India and the Middle East. It has been used for centuries in traditional ayurvedic medicine due to its robust healing properties. Modern research has revealed numerous health benefits of Boswellia, from reducing inflammation to relieving pain. Inflammation is the body's natural response to injury or infection, but chronic inflammation can lead to a host of health issues. Research has shown that Boswellia's active compounds, called boswellic acids, have powerful anti-inflammatory properties that can help reduce inflammation. In one study, participants with rheumatoid arthritis experienced a significant decrease in their inflammation after taking Boswellia supplements. Pain is another common issue that Boswellia can help with. Studies have shown that Boswellia can help reduce pain associated with conditions such as osteoarthritis, menstrual cramps, and headaches. This is likely due to its anti-inflammatory effects, as well as its ability to reduce the production of certain pain-causing chemicals in the body. Boswellia may also help improve respiratory health. Studies have shown that Boswellia can reduce the symptoms of asthma, such as wheezing and shortness of breath. It is thought that this is due to its anti-inflammatory effects, which can reduce inflammation in the airways. Boswellia can also help improve digestive health. It has been shown to reduce intestinal inflammation and improve the health of the digestive system. This can help improve digestion, reduce bloating, and reduce symptoms of irritable bowel syndrome. Finally, Boswellia may be beneficial for the immune system. Its anti-inflammatory properties can help reduce inflammation in the body, which can help the immune system work more efficiently. Additionally, Boswellia has been shown to boost the activity of immune cells, which can help the body fight off infections more effectively. Overall, Boswellia is a powerful herb with numerous health benefits. It has been used for centuries in traditional ayurvedic medicine and modern research has revealed its potential for reducing inflammation, relieving pain, and improving respiratory, digestive, and immune health.

Brahmi

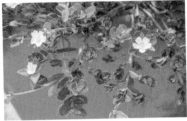

Brahmi, also known as Bacopa Monnieri, is an Ayurvedic herb that has been used for centuries in traditional Indian medicine. It is believed to have a variety of health benefits. It is known for its ability to improve cognitive function, reduce stress and anxiety, improve memory, and boost the immune system. Brahmi is an adaptogenic herb, meaning it helps the body adapt to stress and to maintain balance in the body. It is known to have a calming effect on the mind, as well as helping to reduce anxiety and depression. It also helps to balance hormones and regulate mood swings, which can be beneficial for those with PMS and menopause. Brahmi is also known to improve cognitive function and memory. It has been studied extensively and has been found to improve alertness, mental clarity, and the ability to learn and remember new information. It has also been found to have a positive effect on the brain's neurotransmitters, which can help with dementia, Alzheimer's disease, and other age-related cognitive decline. Brahmi is also known to improve the immune system by increasing the production of white blood cells, which help fight off infection and disease. It is also known to help reduce inflammation, which is beneficial for those suffering from arthritis and other inflammatory conditions. In addition to these health benefits, Brahmi may also be beneficial for those with diabetes, high cholesterol, and high blood pressure. It has been studied for its effects on blood sugar levels and cholesterol and has been found to have a positive effect. Overall, Brahmi is an incredible herb that has many health benefits. It can help improve cognitive function, reduce stress and anxiety, improve memory, and boost the immune system. It can also help regulate hormones, reduce inflammation, and even have a beneficial effect on diabetes, cholesterol, and blood pressure. For these reasons, Brahmi is an amazing herb to incorporate into your daily health regimen.

Liquorice Root

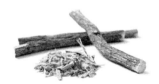

Liquorice root is a natural and powerful herbal remedy that has been used for centuries to treat a variety of ailments. The root of the liquorice plant is where the medicinal benefits of the herb originate. It is commonly used in teas, dietary supplements, and topical applications. Liquorice root is packed with active compounds and vitamins that are beneficial for overall health and well-being. One of the most notable health benefits of liquorice root is its anti-inflammatory properties. The active ingredient in liquorice root, glycyrrhizin, has been found to reduce inflammation in the body. This can be beneficial for those suffering from arthritis, gout, and other inflammatory conditions. Liquorice root also has antioxidant properties which can help protect against free radical damage and oxidative stress. This can help improve overall health and may even help slow the aging process. Liquorice root is also known for its anti-viral properties. It has been used to treat ailments such as colds, flu, and even the common cold. It is believed to be effective against certain viruses, such as the herpes virus, which can cause cold sores. Liquorice root is also believed to be beneficial for digestive health. It has been used to treat stomach ulcers, acid reflux, and other digestive problems. It can also help improve the absorption of nutrients and minerals. Liquorice root has also been found to be beneficial for the skin. It has anti-bacterial, anti-fungal, and anti-inflammatory properties which can help reduce redness and swelling, while also improving skin tone and texture. In addition to the health benefits of liquorice root, it has also been used for its potential to improve mood and reduce stress. Studies have found that liquorice root can help reduce feelings of anxiety and depression. Overall, liquorice root is a natural and powerful herbal remedy that can provide a range of health benefits. From reducing inflammation to improving skin health, liquorice root can be a great addition to any natural health regimen.

Gotu Kola

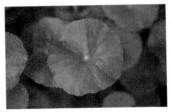

Gotu Kola, also known as Centella Asiatica, is an herb that has been used in traditional Chinese and Ayurvedic medicine for centuries. It is known for its wide range of health benefits, including improved mental clarity and focus, improved digestion, and improved circulation. Gotu Kola is a source of several essential vitamins and minerals, including Vitamin C, Vitamin A, and Vitamin B6. It also contains essential fatty acids and phytonutrients. Studies have found that these nutrients can help improve mental clarity and focus and may even reduce anxiety and depression. Additionally, the herb is known for its anti-inflammatory and antioxidant properties, both of which can help reduce inflammation and protect the body from oxidative damage. Gotu Kola is also known for its ability to improve circulation and digestion. Studies have shown that the herb can help reduce inflammation in the veins, which can lead to improved circulation. Additionally, the herb has been shown to improve digestion by increasing the production of digestive enzymes. This can help to improve nutrient absorption and reduce digestive discomfort. Another benefit of Gotu Kola is its potential to help heal wounds. Studies have found that the herb can help to speed up wound healing, reduce inflammation, and reduce scarring. Finally, Gotu Kola has been found to have potential anti-aging effects. Studies have shown that the herb can help to reduce wrinkles and improve skin elasticity. It can also help to reduce the appearance of age spots, discoloration, and other signs of aging. Overall, Gotu Kola is an incredibly powerful herb that can offer a wide range of health benefits. It is best taken as part of a healthy diet and lifestyle and should be used alongside other natural remedies for the best results.

Bitter Melon

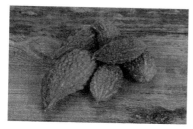

Bitter melon (Momordica charantia) is a unique vegetable with a range of health benefits. It is a tropical and subtropical vine native to parts of Asia, Africa, and the Caribbean, and has been used in traditional medicine for centuries as a folk remedy for a variety of ailments. Bitter melon has many beneficial nutrients, including vitamins A, B1, B2, C, iron, potassium, magnesium, and zinc. It is also a good source of dietary fibre. One of the most notable health benefits of bitter melon is its potential to reduce blood sugar levels. Studies have shown that bitter melon extract can reduce blood glucose levels by up to 30%, making it a potential treatment for type 2 diabetes. Bitter melon can also help to reduce cholesterol levels, improve insulin sensitivity, and reduce inflammation. Bitter melon has also been found to have potential anti-cancer properties. Studies have shown that it can help to inhibit the growth of cancer cells and reduce tumour size. It is also believed to have antioxidant and anti-inflammatory properties, which can help to protect against a variety of diseases and illnesses. Bitter melon can be consumed in a variety of ways, including raw, cooked, or as a supplement. It is important to note that the vegetable can have a very bitter taste, so it may be best to mix it with other foods or beverages to reduce the taste. In conclusion, bitter melon is a unique vegetable with a range of health benefits. It is a rich source of beneficial nutrients and has been shown to reduce blood sugar levels, reduce cholesterol levels, and potentially have anti-cancer properties. It can be consumed in a variety of ways and may be best mixed with other foods or beverages to reduce its bitter taste.

SPECIAL MENTIONS

Sulforaphane

Sulforaphane is a compound found in cruciferous vegetables like broccoli and cabbage, as well as in broccoli sprouts. It has been shown to have a number of health benefits, including anti-cancer properties, antioxidant benefits, and anti-inflammatory effects. One of the most notable benefits of sulforaphane is its potential anti-cancer effects. Studies have found that it can inhibit the growth of certain cancer cells and reduce tumour size. It may also help to protect DNA from damage and reduce cell death. Additionally, it can help to enhance the body's natural ability to fight cancer cells. Sulforaphane also has antioxidant properties, which can help to protect the body from oxidative stress. Oxidative stress can damage cells and lead to a number of health conditions, such as heart disease, diabetes, and cancer. Sulforaphane can help to neutralize free radicals in the body, which can help to reduce the risk of these conditions. In addition, sulforaphane has anti-inflammatory effects. It can help to reduce inflammation in the body, which can help to reduce the risk of certain diseases. Studies have found that it can reduce inflammation in the skin, joints, and respiratory system. It can also help to reduce inflammation in the gut, which may help to reduce the risk of digestive disorders. Broccoli sprouts are a good source of sulforaphane and have been found to have even more concentrated levels of the compound than mature broccoli. Studies have found that they can help to reduce inflammation in the gut, reduce oxidative stress, and protect DNA from damage. They have also been found to have anti-cancer effects and can help to reduce tumour size. In conclusion, sulforaphane and broccoli sprouts have a number of health benefits. They can help to reduce inflammation, protect DNA from damage, and reduce the risk of certain diseases. They may also have anti-cancer effects and can help to reduce tumour size. For these reasons, they are a great addition to any healthy diet.

Irish Seamoss

Irish Seamoss, known scientifically as Chondrus crispus, is a species of seaweed that is native to the Atlantic Coast of Europe, Canada, and North America. Seamoss is a nutrient-rich superfood that has been used for centuries as a traditional remedy for a variety of health issues. It is believed to have many health benefits, including boosting the immune system, aiding digestion, and promoting heart health. The most notable health benefit of Irish Seamoss is its high concentration of minerals and nutrients. Seamoss is an excellent source of iodine, potassium, calcium, magnesium, zinc, iron, and manganese. Its high mineral content is believed to be beneficial for the immune system, aiding in the production of white blood cells and improving the body's ability to fight infection. Seamoss is also rich in vitamins A, B, C, and E, which are essential for the body's overall health and wellbeing. Irish Seamoss is also believed to help with digestion. It is known to be a natural laxative, helping to ease constipation and promote regularity. Seamoss is also thought to have anti-inflammatory properties, which can be beneficial in treating a number of gastrointestinal conditions, such as Crohn's disease and ulcerative colitis. Furthermore, Irish Seamoss is believed to be beneficial for the heart, as its high mineral content can help to reduce high blood pressure and cholesterol levels. Finally, Irish Seamoss is believed to be beneficial for the skin. It is rich in antioxidants, which can help to protect the skin from damage caused by free radicals. Additionally, its high mineral content can help to nourish and hydrate the skin, leaving it looking and feeling healthy. In summary, Irish Seamoss is a nutrient-rich superfood that is believed to have many health benefits.

Natto

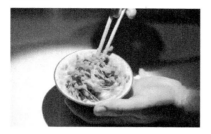

Natto, a traditional Japanese food, has a reputation for being one of the healthiest and most nutritious foods in the world. It is made from fermented soybeans and is a great source of protein, vitamins, minerals, and other beneficial nutrients. Natto is also known for its many health benefits, which include aiding digestion, improving cardiovascular health, and boosting the immune system. One of the main benefits of natto is its high nutritional content. Natto is an excellent source of protein, providing about 10g per serving. It is also rich in essential vitamins and minerals, including vitamins B1, B2, B6, and C, as well as calcium, iron, magnesium, phosphorus, and potassium. Natto also contains a variety of beneficial enzymes that can aid in digestion, as well as probiotics, which can help to maintain a healthy gut. Natto is also known for its cardiovascular benefits. It is a good source of vitamin K2, which is important for maintaining healthy blood vessels and reducing the risk of heart disease. Natto also contains high levels of omega-3 fatty acids, which can help reduce blood pressure and cholesterol levels. Natto is also known for its immune-boosting properties. It contains a variety of antioxidants, which can help to protect the body from free radicals and reduce inflammation. Natto is also a good source of vitamin C, which is important for stimulating the immune system and fighting off infections. Natto is a great addition to any diet, as it is low in calories and packed with beneficial nutrients. It is a great source of protein and essential vitamins and minerals, and its many health benefits make it an excellent choice for anyone looking to improve their overall health.

Fermented foods

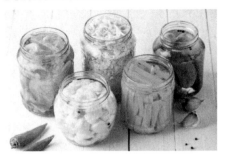

Fermented foods are a traditional part of many diets around the world, but they are gaining popularity in the West as people become more health conscious. Fermented foods are made by a process of lacto-fermentation, which is the same process used to make yogurt, cheese, beer, and wine. This process breaks down the carbohydrates in the food and produces lactic acid, which acts as a preservative and adds flavour to the food. Fermented foods are a great source of probiotics, which are beneficial bacteria that help promote a healthy gut and improve digestion. Sauerkraut is one of the most popular fermented foods and is made from cabbage and salt. It can be eaten plain or as a condiment. Sauerkraut is high in vitamins A, B, and C and is a great source of dietary fibre, which helps promote regularity and can help reduce the risk of certain types of cancer. Sauerkraut is also a good source of probiotics, which can help improve digestion and boost the immune system. Miso is a traditional Japanese fermented food made from soybeans, salt, and koji, a type of fungus. It is a popular ingredient in many Japanese dishes and is often used to flavour soups and sauces. Miso is rich in protein, fibre, vitamins, and minerals, and is a good source of probiotics. It is also believed to help reduce inflammation and improve heart health. Kimchi is a fermented food made from cabbage, radish, or other vegetables, and it is a staple in Korean cuisine. It is typically served as a side dish or a condiment and is high in vitamins and minerals. Kimchi is also rich in probiotics, which can help improve digestion and boost the immune system. In conclusion, fermented foods are an excellent source of probiotics and other nutrients, and they can be a great addition to any diet. They are easy to make at home, and they can add flavour and nutrition to a variety of dishes. They are also believed to have numerous health benefits, including improved digestion, boosted immunity, and reduced inflammation. So, if you're looking for a way to get more nutrition from your meals, try incorporating some fermented foods into your diet.

Green Tea

Green tea has been consumed for centuries in many different cultures, and its popularity continues to rise in modern times. This is because green tea has numerous health benefits that make it a great choice for anyone seeking to improve their health and wellness. One of the best known benefits of green tea is its high antioxidant content. Antioxidants are powerful compounds that help protect cells from damage caused by free radicals, which can lead to chronic diseases like cancer. Green tea is loaded with polyphenols, which are powerful antioxidants that can help protect against cell damage. Studies have also shown that drinking green tea can help reduce the risk of heart disease, stroke, and other cardiovascular diseases. Green tea is also rich in catechins, which are compounds that can help reduce inflammation and the risk of certain diseases. Studies have found that catechins can help reduce the risk of type 2 diabetes, obesity, and some forms of cancer. Green tea also contains theanine, an amino acid that can help reduce stress and improve mental focus. In addition, green tea is a natural source of caffeine, which can help improve energy levels, focus, and concentration. It also contains vitamins and minerals, including vitamins A, C, and E, as well as potassium and magnesium. All of these nutrients can help support overall health and wellness. Finally, green tea can help aid digestion and weight loss. Studies have shown that green tea can help boost metabolism and burn fat, which can help you reach your weight loss goals. Additionally, green tea can help reduce bloating and improve overall digestive health. Overall, green tea is an incredibly healthy beverage that can provide numerous benefits. From its antioxidant content to its ability to aid digestion, green tea is a great choice for anyone looking to improve their health.